The Alkaline Miracle Diet

Detox Immunity & Weight-Loss Lifestyle

What it takes to have an Alkaline immune environment flight response to the dangers of disease

Table of Contents

Dedication

I dedicate this book to the pioneer Dr. Sebi, who I learned my research from. To my children who supported me throughout my journey. And to my immediate family. Most of all I thank God for his grace in blessing me.

BACKGROUND

HOW I DISCOVERED THE ALKALINE WEIGHT LOSS PLAN

You'll agree with me that losing significant weight in some areas of the body without affecting our radiance is what we all crave. What do I mean by this? Simple! We all lust for a certain type of food that is injurious to our health. We then justify our actions with the uncertainty of longevity, giving in to the misconception that we never know when we die, you only live once. While this may also be a timeless truth, making healthy decisions on the foods we eat will undoubtedly tune up digestive organs, the skin (largest organ), and nevertheless and overall healthier heart. An unhealthy lifestyle can stumble upon you without no warning that something is going wrong, for example a heart attack. Have I seen cases of a healthy person get an unexpectant illness or disease? Yes, that's because many of the interruptions inside our body is beyond our control. There are plenty of skilled surgeons who could vouch for the shortcomings in saving lives. Just reflect as a kid growing up, all the excessive food, parties, dinners, and snacks consumed over a decade or two. When you get to a certain age, the body has worked tremendously hard to get to where it is. Although our body is built like a machine, the fluids still need to be flushed.

As we age, lowering the heavy maintenance of our digestive system is our first step. This is important because essentially our energy to burn fat tends to decrease the older, we get.

However, it can be easily increased with regular cardio fitness with intermittent fasting. Which is why, I want to share with you the details of this journey. Because when something malfunctions in the body knowing what to replace at maximum intake is not a temporary fast operation. The quality of this book walks you through how I readjusted my internal environment to a more conscious control of reducing unhealthy free radicals. Making a permanent commitment to eat only alkaline foods became my lifestyle? Lifestyle is simply the way we optimize what we do for ourselves daily. An all-day alkaline detox ois what this diet consists of.

A readjusted living of what to eat, how fast does this work for my body, how will this benefit me, how long should I eat this way? If you think about it, this matches the same criteria we ask ourselves on daily spending or other longevity decisions like life insurance. Life Insurance costs are much lenient with a person at maximum health. If you take an extensive look at the health insurance bills, you'd come to the inevitable conclusion that a reckless eating or bad habit has a major relation to shortening an individual's lifespan. Not to mention finding the right life insurance company to honor your policy. A miracle diet is not easy, it's a collection of power alkaline foods for a better body composition to wellness. An all-organic body detox and meal guide regime that can go with any schedule. As most of us have multiple tasks, eating on the go has become more fluent. Working at home is easier than it seems when your able to avoid distractions. Imagine focusing on improving your health and you see your co-worker walk past with pizza or fried chicken. Instantly your brain sensory tries to take over your thoughts. It is also my hope that after you finish reading this book, you will have the blueprint of an alkaline organic natural antioxidant radiance.

Common misconceptions, most people fail on diets. Two reasons, the fear of the impossibilities of reaching their goal and relapse. It is very compelling to flush out all the toxins for a specific health problem, especially if you're were born with a complex disease. For instance, an auto immune disease is forever, but it didn't stop me from seeking a salvation for a stronger body. And for a natural look, the goal tends to seem never-ending. Mainly because losing weight can ignite anxiety. An anticipation of faster results. Perhaps, you have a nice look, and you'd rather a natural toned appearance and increase immunity instead of constant cosmetic surgery and adjustments. This was my premise of seeking an all-organic antioxidant diet to stay on. And if you abuse alcohol and nicotine for 20 years, it's time to retract to prevent any further damage. The damage we cause to our insides will begin to appear on the outside. All parallel to the transition into a healthier lifestyle. I had to tell myself in the mirror daily, not to be conjoined with the myriads of people who failed at commitment. Preparing what to eat the day before became a job, to a living dream. Coming from a common place today that many of us resort to eating foods we like, instead of what we need. What we like sounds better if you're a healthy kid. Yet, when its' time to detox the internal organs, knowing what foods to eat and what it does to fix or repair health issues doesn't matter the age.

Our body can detox areas where disease and cancer are said to be unable to thrive with natural foods found in our earth. Though this has not been conducted in a laboratory. I gathered extensive research from the study of Dr. Sebi's philosophy of alkaline foods. I also extended research about processed and GMO foods.

You must ask yourself why? For the most part anything that must be proven has to be conducted in a laboratory with a test of a live individual to experiment. This is not to mislead you. This is not a miracle of a cure. Nor will this be costly, rather designed to cut back you're spending on unhealthy expensive or cheap foods. To affordable, antioxidant (bacteria fighting) meals, an investment that will aid in the process of naturally cleansing your colon, digestive organ, skin, and detox. At the same time shedding out my weakened cells.

So, let's start from the beginning. I first would like to say switching to a permanent lifestyle was not easy to adapt. I had to crutch my thoughts. Focusing on staying strong and not giving up.

"Sometimes you have to go through something in order to grow from something".

It came without notice, however, if I knew what to anticipate, I could have possibly relapsed without witnessing and went a different direction in life. Thank goodness I didn't!

I was in a relationship with a man who had complete control over the way I felt about myself. Abuse was daily both mentally and physically. Exhausted from seeking help of family and friends, I felt unworthy, In other words, I ate recklessly, I consumed alcohol, and smoked cigarettes to cope with the feeling of hopelessness. Disappointed in myself for being in fear and allowing him to mistreat me. He knew I had no one to intervene the relationship safely. I felt less and less of a person, becoming numb to pain and silent to happiness. Until one day all it took was a split-second decision which ended it all and soon became a miraculous aftermath. I can remember screaming inside my head, desiring to break free as tears fell down the sides of my emotionless face. I rise seeking to seize the day to free myself from painful memories. Scanning my brain from the past, what I needed to do to be happy with myself. I laid supine, drained but motionlessly awakened, I sat on the edge of my bed. My body and my mental health ultimately felt disconnected. Convincing myself, today I was going to come up with a solution.

I kept feeling hesitation of uncertainty. I have nowhere to go and no one to turn to, no one I could hide out with to reinvent myself. I couldn't think about anything eventful besides breathing the smell of traveling wind and smiling. Looking out the window in the bedroom after brushing my teeth and washing my face. I watched the heavy lowered clouds with no precipitation hoover away to lighten the day. Feeling the sensation that I just needed to leave the house to simply go for an afternoon ride to try to clear my head. I needed to regain focus on goals and dreams. There was zero trust in the relationship, but we stayed together to be parents. Fed up with walking on eggshells, I change into some sweatpants, swiftly gathering my personal things like you know lip gloss, ID. Shifting out the bedroom in seconds towards the living room. I hear his cell phone ring. I knew in a few he is going to use the bathroom.

In one motion I reach to open the front door. Due to the weak nails in the anchor of the front door, once I opened the screen door my cover was blown. In an autonomous motion I hurriedly close the screen door. Before leaving, I left a message (sticky note) written "I was going for a ride" on the bathroom mirror, hoping he would read it after I left out the door and got in the car at least. Basically, I wanted to avoid an altercation or argument by leaving and where would I be going. I wanted to avoid being manipulated with attachment and control is all I could think once I got in the car. Hurrying with a speed walk to my car. I could hear behind me the front screen door open. I immediately hear him coming to stop me. Suddenly, my arm is grabbed fiercely from behind. At that moment my heartbeat in my ear paused.

As I turn around, looking up to a six-foot two man, I see the redness in his eye of enrage in slow motion. He says to me in one breath of each sentence, minus syllables, "You're not leaving this house, where are you going to go? You have no friends". Manipulating me to feel hopeless. From that point, my desire to leave gets the best of me. I yank my arm firmly from his grip, suddenly I feel a sense of pride. I say back, "So what I have no friends, let me go or I'll call the cops!" All I remember was the last sound of the alphabet in the word cops echo to mute. I couldn't believe for the first time I lost consciousness. I somehow stumble back sliding down along the side back door of my vehicle, like a boxer getting knocked out and falling back on the rope. Except I didn't get a chance to protect myself.

In the worst pain imaginable, I woke up from my twelve-year-old daughter lifting my face from the rocky car port. Everything sounded muffled. Nothing in me could ever hurt my memory more than this moment. Frightened, I could feel her hands shaking while trying to open my eyes. Sounding broken, hearing my child cry to me. Panicky asks, "Mommy! Are you okay? Please get up", muffled in my ear, all the sound I could hear as my own child guided to my feet. I began to slowly stand up. Seeing blood dripping out my mouth, my face stinging in pain, my child crying and rubbing my arms to awaken me to consciousness. As my eyesight came to focus, I became clear of what just happened. Horrified and embarrassed, I couldn't look at my daughter in the eyes. I was in too much pain in the face. I knew something was broken. Silently muttering to my child, "Don't let anything happen to your brother. Don't let anyone take off with him, and I will be back!". Not caring where he ran too, hoping he knew I could never forgive another, "I'm sorry, I didn't mean it,". I knew from the deep burning pain in my face, I needed a doctor. I head to the ER. As I'm trying to drive in agony, I realize I needed to be accompanied for support.

With the unbearable pain getting worse, there was no way I could turn back from being afraid. So, in this case, I didn't. I head to my closest friend last known location, locate his whereabouts immediately from his closest relative, who knew where he was at. He wasn't the type of guy to keep a phone on, yet still loyal. The relative notified him of the urgency, so he was already waiting for me outside, when I arrived. He takes over driving so I could bring myself to. For all I could think of on the way to the ER was getting back to my kids and hoping the damage wasn't severe. Scared to look in the mirror at myself on the way to the hospital, tears dried to my cheeks. As we arrive, barely able to move my mouth, I get out first to check in and head to be seated.

The patients waiting to be seen in the lobby stare awkwardly at my face. Praying no one would remember me. I no longer could cry the pain was just too unbearable. I bury my face in my homeboys' comfort as he waited with me. Only for a short time, he kept feeling he would be accused of injuring me, so he caught a ride home, when I headed back to be seen. Meanwhile the personal responsible could still be at the house doing God knows what. I knew however, I was in no shape to do anything besides getting care. I wasn't surprised this happened, I blamed myself. I should have got away sooner. I believed the man responsible was supposed to be a person I would never let anything happened to his son, so why harm me? There was only one answer to that as I boldly stayed in my mind. It didn't take long to be seen, and before you know it, the X-ray came back identifying a broken jaw. I sustained a fracture to both sides of my lower jaw along with the infamous sharp stabbing pain to my face. Sedated while waiting for further instructions, when I woke up, I was given a referral, instructions and numbing medication liquid Hydrocodone, until a surgeon could reconstruct my jaw.

I left unable to feel anything mentally and physically, completely numb. Permanently shattered, emotionally and physically delicate from a traumatic experience. I was in severe pain from morning to sleep, after surgery and the recovery was pure torture. My teeth were wired shut. The recovery consisted of a liquid diet which was my only choice to eat for 6 weeks with no instruction or nutrition manual. Just about every morning and evening, in the first week, I would do nothing but cry. Being unable to open my teeth for air. I hardly had the air to cry for long. I found it useful to just lay down and let my tears just fall. Using the liquid hydrocodone to hurry the thoughts away. Having no clue at first as too what to eat felt like I was in a psychiatric jacket. How will I survive? How will I eat? The first week I just sipped on liquid hydrocodone and ensure.

Experiencing night sweats, going in and out of mental breakdowns, at the end of the first week I rapidly lost weight, I got wrapped into the assessment to research other liquid foods and so on to healthy nutrition to keep muscle. I became hooked, creating a liquid meal for every two hours I had to consume. Majority of everything I blended was an organically blended, except ensures and regular tomato, potato, mushroom, and organic broth soup. I basically survived, throughout the day for 6 weeks consuming liquid only. I had lost tremendous weight throughout all parts of my body over the 6 weeks of liquid only.

Which did not include cardio, mainly because I couldn't control my breathing with my teeth wire shut. The 7th week was a dawdling readjustment with slow, steady steps to eating solid soft foods, almost like eating baby food. Despite the liberty to finally resurface to open my jaw to eat, I still could not consume large amounts of food and open my mouth wide. Still to this day, I still can't. The entire recovery of 7 weeks was composed of a restricted liquid to soft diet the last week. It was torture at first to incorporate a liquid meal every 2 hours. But once I got my brain on schedule, I was at the beginning of a new lifestyle. It would have been nice to have a care assistance or someone at that time to assist me with my recovery, but unfortunately, healthcare was complicated in my country and no way could I burden my oldest child or younger child. The significance of this journey was the light bulb that pushed me to dig deeper in my research for organic blended liquid meals and other vitamin full nutrition. I began studying the quantity of rich vitamins and the purpose it serves in the bodies cytoplasmic process, secondhandedly, I began researching the teachings of Dr. Sebi's organic antioxidant alkaline food research. I captioned where to find the vegetation of alkaline foods, how to properly prep and cook without dehydrating the antioxidants. Informed on how to prep food and thus eliminating saturated and animal fat. I still needed healthy mono and polyunsaturated fat to keep protein. During my liquid diet, I would drink vanilla ensures for protein.

Today of course, I intermittently maintain a liquid diet with rotation of solid alkaline vegetables and fasting. I prepare my vegetables in three ways. Steam, lightly boil, or skillet with monosaturated and polyunsaturated fat oil. Dr. Sebi s' diet restricted indigestion of any preserved meat and the blood of animals inside the body, which I was not able to consume anyway during my injury and after. If you think about the life expectancy of animals regardless of unfortunate events, they are living in the outdoor terrain of a compromised plantation.

Which is a reason why the popularity of plant-based food is on the rise. Animals are over-crowded in their habitat by the day. Soon there will be more plant-based restaurants or on the menu at traditional restaurants. Honestly, maybe even fast-food plant- based franchises. When you think about the habitat of the animals that are sold in groceries, where they sleep, what they eat, do they get ticks or mosquito bites, do they get colds or diseases too? It's too much on the body to fight, not to mention other leading causes of a shorter life expectancy. Realizing the significant change in my skin and weight from a liquid diet with no meat, I could see the truth. Saddened by the falsely hood of eating animals throughout my childhood, I now learned that I was eating everything the animal suffered throughout their lifetime. I lost my appetite. Taking account, if the animal was ever sad or angry, is the lifestyle I versioned. I am what I eat is a truthful motto. I stargazed and reflected on everything I have ate that wasn't any good. I realized the hard way that I was not eating right. As I look back recovering from my injury, I overcame the unbearable pain of not being able to open my mouth and eat, invigorating to blending tomato juices, banana juices, milk blends and mashed potatoes to survive. Not just for a day but for several weeks. Into a now incorporating an advanced antioxidant alkaline environment because of what I am now fighting. A new lifestyle, a new way to live.

The most difficult part of changing to a liquid diet was that I first had to drink through a straw inserting the front on the side to the very back wall of my mouth, as close to my throat as possible. I also was currently enrolled in college during this hard time, which was a private college very strict on attendance. If I stayed home to recover, I would have had to re-do the courses. Meaning I wouldn't graduate in time. Another impact, I was not willing to surrender to, as I am moments away from betterment, I disconnect what anyone would say and just went to school anyway. I took notes or wrote notes to my instructors if I needed to communicate. It was the worse feeling having the same facial expression, unable to smile. Every day, I would mark off each completed day on the calendar as if I was soon to be released from prison. I brushed the front of my teeth 3 times a day with baking soda. In addition, I had to have a professional teeth cleaning inside and throughout my mouth after the wires were removed from my teeth. After the recovery of my injury, the 8th week, I dove into overeating anything soft to eat. I consumed ice cream, macaroni and cheese, cheese grits, French fries, donuts, etc. Eating two bigger meals a day and added saturated fat from chips and cookies, I gained 10 pounds in just 3 weeks. Labored with feelings of sadness from overcoming my injury for some reason, I can't explain why I desperately ate after now I'm proportionately slim. It's important to recognize the reaction the body yields when it lacks certain nutrients and cravings. It can suddenly relapse. Essentially, is what I mentally overpowered from living on a liquid diet for 6 weeks and soft foods for the 7th week but now I had to overcome temptation with consciousness.

In Starting the Routine chapter, I break down how to begin preparing alkaline foods to blend. The struggle during a liquid diet lifestyle change was largely my mental, going from eating what I use to eat, eating to what I could only eat, to adjusting from temptation and influence. Researching as many liquid drinks as possible I could make a day was tedious. A liquid diet for 7 weeks is a natural liposuction so to speak. Looking back at how much damage I use to recklessly eat heavy fried foods, numerous alcoholic episodic introverted retreats to escape pain, was the reason for my fat gain and low immunity.

I now became stronger to the resistance of eating bad food mentally and internally experiencing an all or nothing liquid alkaline diet.

Bad foods I need to mention like eating deep fried chicken, turkey, pork, etc., butter downed with cheese or high sugar, maple high fructose syrup or over spiced seasoned entrees, I couldn't consume ever again. Replacing all these meats with mushrooms, plant-based meat, organic honey, antioxidant seasoning and less sugar.

I appeared naturally toned with vibrant skin on a liquid diet. My body didn't resemble a sizzle of saturated or animal fat. Saturated and animal fat in the past before my injury, would make my jaw have a double roll underneath. Nonetheless, the hardest fat to eliminate overall was my belly fat called Visceral fat. My tummy and waist were completely slim. Visceral fat will attach around the abdominal organs deep inside the lower cavity of the body. Even if you have a small stomach visceral fat attaches in the organs. This becomes the fat your body doesn't need. It can initiate problems in the body, for example: high blood-pressure, diabetes, stroke, high cholesterol swelling, and other circulatory issues. However, my results were results of a teenage body but healthy.

So, here's when my journey gets serious for me, after I went through my harrowing injury and post-injury phase, I went in for a routine check-up after. It was scheduled two months after my injury, which gave me enough time to readjust, well kindly leaving out the mental ups and downs after the 8th week recovering, I overate in foods I knew were unhealthy. When my physician walked in the room, it was at first glance, looking at me, did he discover my neck enlarged abnormally, quickly asking if I was ever told I may have goiter. He examined my physical appearance, put in tests for my blood and concluded to me, "I may have to send you in for further testing and an ultrasound on your neck". He states until then, he will know for certain the cause of my swollen neck. I go to complete my labs and return to another scheduled visit, he goes over the results and says, "It appears you have what is called Graves' Disease". We tested your hormones and other lab work, and the symptoms are caused from something you are eating or is hereditary. Which is causing an imbalance and over-production of hormones. It was then immediately did I know I really had to stop eating bad food. He then puts in an appointment to be made for an ultrasound of my neck to look at my thyroid. It was scheduled. So, I later go in for more blood work and the ultrasound of the neck. The results from the ultrasound were mailed to me, indicating that I have Hyperthyroidism and a small tumor in my neck. Even my ankles and legs were swollen which was a symptom I was experiencing when I ate bad foods. And here I was thinking I was getting cuter by getting thicker. Dr. goes over the management of being on medication to take daily for the Graves' Disease and that I would need to be rescheduling to see if the tumor is growing in 6 months to return.

With the combination of diagnosis of an auto immune disorder, a previous herniated disk and sciatica damage from a past injury, a fractured jaw and now a benign tumor, I was in devastation to following up for regular visits. What job is going to allow me to go to numerous Dr. visits, is what I negatively judged myself with. But within realistic capacity, most employers can't afford excessive missed days. I needed to be unweeding from eating unhealthy food to back to no meat, no preservatives, no saturated fat, little to no calorie diet. Forced and awaken by the premise to fight for my life it was my new destiny to overcome my autoimmune disease.

This was the churning into this new profound miracle of alkaline foods. Something to work around the clock naturally to work inside to flush out toxins inside my body. In an alkaline environment, subjective complaints tend to dilute precedence from animal consumption and saturated fat in short time. For instance, my skin tightened reducing the sagging of my skin. I was beginning to feel less sluggish. From being on a previous liquid diet, I had the potential to recreate an alkaline environment that would be hard for disease to mingle or hide especially cells involved in the suppression of my auto immune disorder. Invariably allowing my body's immunity to easily spot infected cells by outnumbering them with healthy cells. First, I had to detox out the bad, dead, unwanted, and unhealthy cells. Starting every morning on an empty stomach, to impact my guts the hardest with an alkaline antioxidant drink. Since your skin is the largest organ in the body, the skin ultimately begins to appear *environmental-free* after the detox process begins. Other's close to me could see a change in my skin's radiance my complexion appeared lighter, youthful, and younger. I didn't have to apply much make-up. My skin contained a natural organic youthful glow from detoxing better that going through an Esthetician. My new appearance displayed a reverse in my age, in which people mistake me regularly as a decade younger even still to this day. I must admit, I did look my age before my jaw fractured. In fact, after many mistaken concepts of my age, my research and commitment to eating alkaline foods only was now proof I needed to document and share my truth about alkaline foods.

Holistically, this weight loss journey is more complex than any competition. For instance, not too many people will believe that what you were born and taught to eat is bad to the chemistry in the cells of your body. It is my opinion, if not hereditary health related, eating, and consuming meat and blood of animals is the reason for acidity and less immunity in the body. In other words, dependence on man-made medication to speed up the results. There are many controversial diets and powdered drinks that in my belief are not strictly alkaline antioxidant food. Nothing against the powdered drinks it's just its man-made if not grown from the ground. It's neither not a grown alkaline antioxidant, powdered man-made substance or could contain traces of meat. You see, if you put nothing but consistent alkaline antioxidants in your body on a well-timed basis, you are only increasing the detox of bad fat, unhealthy cells to be weakened and expunged out the body through either perspiration or colon. Cardio, I incorporate as a fast-working toxin remover. Underneath the skin is another place saturated fat tends to hide. Thus, combining cardio with an all-antioxidant diet for a maximum detox.

Antioxidants are what we need to inhibit oxidation of free radicals that may damage the cells of organisms in the body. Ascorbic acid from eating meat may inhibit or decrease the compounds that are needed to inhibit oxidation. Animals was not going to help me live longer, not to mention when you think about it, animals have a shorter lifespan than humans. Consuming their blood just goes straight throughout one of the most valuable transmission of nutrients in the body which is my stomach and to my colon. The stomach mainly breaks down everything for digestion into the bloodstream and the colon is all that's left of. Inside the colon fecal matter is always being deposited. This is because fecal matter is composed of metabolic waste and epithelial cells in the intestines. Therefore, constant detoxing is important when it comes to the colon. Inside the large intestine water and salts are used to transform waste into a solid mass. The small intestine is to absorb the nutrients by breaking down to rid unnecessary components. Alkaline antioxidants being absorbed continuously throughout the most important manufacture of nutrient absorbent in the digestive process, is when the miracle of prevention occurred for me.

Everything I ate became and was crystal-clear to me and my body - what was in it, how it was made, how it got to where I bought it from, and how much antioxidants is in it? I delivered myself through the test of temptation. The test to reducing the need for pills to control my hormones and Graves' Disease and ultimately reducing my benign tumor. I needed a pellucid simplicity on making the best decision about what I eat to live versus what I live to eat, which I wouldn't judge as 'bad', after all. It was just my idea of being responsible - mirroring a Spartan's self-discipline. If I want to become stronger, I needed to consume the strongest. I visioned the number of vitamins, minerals, and antioxidants I needed to consume daily to keep my body in an alkaline environment. Contrary to constantly eating 3 or 2 big meals a day, working against my immunity reducing the wear and tear in the colon, replacing with one alkaline meal a day instead. The rest would be nothing but snacks of antioxidants.

To say the least, an alkaline environment levitated my body's natural defense with a constant cleanse to my digestive system, stomach, skin, and organs. The unsaturated and saturated fat that was hidden in my organs I had to work off with cardio for faster results. Infused with energy, cardio became the quickest 30-minute fat burn and skin firming, liberating activity for me. It was either I jogged for thirty minutes and stretched 4 times a week or went to the elliptical for 30 minutes and stretched. In between, I would strengthen my shoulders, arms, abdomen, and leg muscles. This whole lifestyle was synonymous to limiting the consumption of daily prescription medications. Even though, there are diseases that we ultimately cannot avoid, this journey effectively presented results for me to rely less on prescription for the smallest cold. It was a devil in disguise, a traumatic injury to recovering only the richest intake of antioxidant my body can take. So, after taking this leap of faith in what natural foods manufacture an alkaline body, for a decade now, my results and experience is truthful. I want you to see how much and what I ate to maximize the oxidation of healthier cellular process in my body.

Introduction

What to expect with the Alkaline Miracle Diet Detox Immunity & Weight Loss Lifestyle Plan?

The Alkaline Miracle Diet is a unique, pulsating experience that I have systematically researched to relieve my illness of Graves' Disease, a tumor in my throat and to alleviate pain misfunctioning of my digestive system in my body. I have meticulously delineated the details of this journey and it doesn't matter if you have a regular no work routine or a full-time job, this detox weight loss plan will not send you to the bathroom. The first things I noticed on the first day was a change in my bowel. I experienced no hesitation to use the bathroom and it came out a lot smoother in weightless. Then gradually, I would begin to see the complexion of my skin appear purified and naturally shiny. I began to have less mucous buildup in my throat and sinus. My skin began to drastically wrap healthier to my muscles and bones. Every day I was noticing the circumference of my love handles and waist inversely shrink to form around the waist and hip. I was also increasing burning fat during crunches or sit-ups occasionally during the week. Overall, I included 30 minutes of cardio 4 times a week. Ascending to the most problematic and premise for this journey was for my body to build up antioxidant immunity to overcome my benign tumor from incinerating to malignant and other inflammations or diseased cells.

Although the switch into this lifestyle was unexpected, the chapters of this book portray an easy seamless transition from acidity to an alkaline antioxidant high protonic internal alkaline environment. When in an alkaline state my disease destructive cells in my cytoplasm react slower inside cell membranes and therefore turn into waste material. Exiting out of my body from cardio and regular bowel. Antioxidants inside the cytoplasm maintain a high concentration of oxidation inside the body. Leading to the removal of wasted cancerous cells out of the cytoplasm and out to the colon, to assign a healthier platform for healthier cells to function healthier. Essentially, when I began replacing high amounts of oxygenated antioxidants into my bloodstream, I was compressing clots and buildup in my circulatory system. For health concerns like, high blood pressure and stroke issues, the circulatory containing platelets, red and white blood cells that are responsible for circulation throughout the body, it is important to maintain a complete blood count. Because this is what will be tested if you have a stroke or cancer. High red blood cells can cause stroke. Ensuring my circulatory system was constantly prespring out toxins to pump healthier blood more efficiently throughout my body, I constantly fasted for several hours of the day, did a little cardio if possible, by the end of the day and drank plenty of alkaline detox.

Understanding first our bodies immunity, must recognize the difference between its' own cells and foreign pathogens. Our immunity is based off several cells that play an important role. T cells have a central role in our body's immunity. T cells are a subtype of white blood cells. When I increase my white blood cells by fasting, eating alkaline food consistently for over a period, increasing detox with cardio, is how the process of acidic body becomes alkaline. Alkalinity is when the body's acidic pH is reduced, it lowers the chances of cancer cells to become more aggressive. An acidic environment only helps cancerous and disease cells spread. Being as though I had a benign tumor in my throat the last thing I wanted to do, was agitate it. I recall a documentary called "What the heck", based on a documentary of major fast-food retailers that are aware that much of their food caused cancer. Although in that movie, none provided a statement, it was the documentary of facts that was conducted to show the difference in eating a plant-based diet versus a genetically modified ingredient or meat preservative. However, when it comes to dealing with a disease, injury, or illness, what I eat has a lot to do with how fast I will recover. I had to increase my intake of a detox drink almost all day long until the evening. By the evening, I would consume, my one nutritious alkaline antioxidant meal. This meal would be the heaviest antioxidant mixture of them all. If you are thinking I am going to much at this, you must understand this is my life, the only life I will ever know. It's important to me to spend every day eating to live.

Starting the routine

Starting the routine to get an alkaline detox, I first DE synthesized my body from everything for several hours of the day. The very first thing I started putting in my body after fasting was about 4 glasses of water and no meat salads. I would drink water all day with a high concentration of steamed or boiled vegetables. Adding a little flavor of apple cider vinegar to detox. On the second day, beginning when I would first wake up, I would fast for as long as half the day again like the first day, but this time incorporating more antioxidants snacks during the day. In the morning, I continued a pattern to fast the body from everything for almost several hours of the day regularly to have maximum results. If you can, sipping on water throughout the day is ok. The purpose of fasting for several hours is so the body can begin locating fat in the body for energy. Now the process of building immunity begins to produce new healthy white cells. Cause you must remember; I no longer smoke or drink. Once white bloods cells are created, they adjoin the T and B cells to fight off infection. B cells simply mitigate the migration of more antigen specific immunoglobulin production for fighting off invasive pathogens. Essentially, this is part of a very important process for the first part of the day. A detox drink to now expand to an alkaline environment. The purpose of having an alkaline environment is so that my body has a maximum chance of fighting off infection and reducing inflammation in the body. Entailing, whenever a pathogen enters my body, I want to feel as confident as ever, that it won't survive.

After fasting in the early morning, the first detox I start off the day with is a delicious organic green tea - brewed with organic antioxidant sliced organic ginger, or sometimes sliced organic turmeric with blended apple cider vinegar, fresh lemon, and organic honey. I learned the advantages of this drink, literally flushing out the entire digestive process. My throat, esophagus, stomach, small intestines to the large intestines, to the colon and affecting the filtration of the liver and kidneys and spleen detoxes. It filters through my intestinal tract dislodging saturated fat, damaged or unneeded metabolic material out. I did not consume any coffee as an antioxidant and while detoxing because coffee is acidic. I know for many coffee goers it is the aide for their day to begin. The acidity is the kick it gives your body in the morning when you have nothing in your stomach. Replacing this with my detox drink, you must know of the significant betterment of the soothe potency of antioxidants instead of coffee waking up the body. Plus. In my opinion, I believe coffee wrinkles the skin around the eyes.

The benefits of these ingredients are abundant. Ginger is said to reduce the risk of cancer and reduces hunger. Which is a major weight lost gunner. Lemon is a rich Vitamin C that acts as an immune booster when activated with ginger in green tea. Even from quitting smoking nicotine, in the morning it felt as though my lungs became clearer. I had less and less mucous in my throat in the morning. Continuing to not smoke became easier, after I quit, cardio made it hard to sneak a puff of a cigarette. If I did try, it made me feel, look more tired and less active to continue cardio. When quitting smoking cigarettes before jogging during cardio, I first would fast walk for thirty minutes at least 4 times a week, at like a track, around my neighborhood, or mainly gym. I started this first when I quit smoking, I waited for two weeks to initiate progression into jogging. I did this so that I would overwhelm my heart. Smoking cigarettes shrinks the veins and arteries and increases buildup in them, so I wanted to use caution. It was important for me to calculate the actual nicotine craving duration ratio over cardio for thirty minutes equaled to a better balance of social dependency.

Concentrating on my thirty-minute jog or on the elliptical was my way of respiring the nicotine from my lungs, bronchi, my heart, and my brain. I mainly would jog in the morning because it was easier for me to jog without anything in my stomach that would cause a cramp or delay my fat burning for the day. The hardest fat to ever burn is the stomach inner drooping fat, the visceral fat. Visceral fat is the cheddar you cannot see because it hides inside our organs. After having three kids and wanting to have a flatter tummy, to speed things up primarily, I needed cardio to confront the hardest detox which was inside my organs. As caution, localizing the burn in the thoracic and abdomen cavity, was important for me to approach this step because I didn't want to overexert my heart and get dizzy. So, I would always sip on my combined alkaline fruit with just the fruit individually put inside my water bottles to make sure I wouldn't feel exertion. Doing this would also change the color and taste as well to my alkaline water drinks, making it tastier. Meditating and stretching for the evenings would help distract me from the temptation of relapsing back to the old unhealthy me. It helped me conserve applying strength and daydream positivity of more-better ways to prepare antioxidant meals. I didn't want to get bored with eating the same meals a day, objectively, it would deteriorate my ambition. So, I recorded a library of different ways to mix delicious alkaline meals.

Setting this up as a road map stamped a duration to eat and include exercising weekly for a lifestyle change. For example, in public schools, children are given a variety of food to choose from, most children skip over fruit and vegetables. Even when they are in a learning environment aware of their potential. It is just embedded in their lifestyle to eat this way. Same goes for alkaline eating except this is developed to reverse unhealthy food cellular damage. If I completed cardio early in the morning, I would then have my detox drink.

I would drink my combination of alkaline fruit like strawberries, blue berries, aloe, and lemon or my green tea blended with antioxidant ingredients after my morning cardio to put back in healthy organic antioxidants from after detoxing out old cellular damage. My detox drink of green tea ingredients was sliced lemon, apple cider vinegar, ginger, and organic honey. You will have to sip on it to adjust the taste with the organic honey. Sometimes in your produce you can find organic fresh mint to also add in green tea. Mint is rich in Vitamins A and C and is a very vital antioxidant for the colon and to help prevent rectal cancer. Each active antioxidant ingredient I used to detox my throat, chest, and lower body to overwhelmingly stock with Vitamins A through E and K.

Vitamin A

Vitamin A benefits the eye vision. It helps keep brain cells protected and skin with antioxidant properties. They are found in sweet potatoes, pumpkin, greens, pumpkins.

Vitamin B12

Vitamin B 12 is not found in plants. Instead, they are most likely found in seafood. Helps improve the brain and our DNA. DNA is helps maintain healthy reproduction of white blood cells.

Vitamin C

High levels of Vitamin C are maintained in cells and tissues with leukocytes. Leukocytes are white blood cells. Known for its citrus flavor, vitamin c is also a rich antioxidant, that helps protect your immunity from free radicals. Free radicals that buildup and contribute to the health illness, such as cancer.

Vitamin D

Vitamin D protects the bones strength and longevity. It also protects the skin's health. They can be found in mushrooms, seafood, bananas, and oranges.

Vitamin E

Protects the fatty layers around our cells. Creates youthful skin and they are mostly found in avocado, blackberries, raspberries, kiwi, mango, nuts, greens.

Vitamin K

Reduces the risk of heart problems and cancer by facilitating rapid communication between cells. Also improves blood clotting for healthy oxygen.

Ginger

Published in the National Library of Medicine, Pubmed.gov, ginger for many centuries has been used in cooking for treatment of many diseases 2014 Elsevier Inc. Ginger is an ingredient that is known traditionally to deliver a high administration of antioxidant that is regulated to improve learning, memory, and deliver an immunosorbent antioxidant throughout the intestinal tract.

Turmeric

Turmeric has been researched to help the bodies inflammatory response to cancer and breast cancer. After series of extensive findings and research, turmeric fights cancer, Alzheimer's disease, and improve heart health. It is a potent anti-inflammatory and antioxidant. When combined on an empty stomach I endure a much greater response and the highest potency to my body's fight for immunity to my autoimmune disease as the first intake of the day. After all I want my colon to cleansed like waterfall.

Aloe

Aloe is known to normalize the healthy function of intestinal gut bacteria, essentially works as a laxative. Aloe boosts the body's metabolism, accelerates weight loss, and immunity. It contains vitamin C and is also rich in oxidants. Cleansing the liver, bladder, kidneys, and spleen. I add this in some of my alkaline fruit drinks with water on days I want to move out more dead bacteria or viruses in my intestinal tract.

Monosaturated Fats

Considered a Mediterranean diet, adequate intake helps memory, fat burning, weight maintenance, heart health, muscle, and mental health. Mainly found in almond, avocado, peanuts, olive oil, nuts, and seeds.

Omega 3Fats

Prevents disease inducing inflammations and brain function. Found in wild caught salmon, flax seeds, chia seeds, navy beans, tuna, mackerel, walnuts.

Fiber & Gut

Benefits yeast, bacteria, and fungi in the intestinal tract. Helping our bodies draw out the nutrients they need from fiber. Also maintains healthy stool, reducing constipation to occur. Too much all at once can make us constipated. High fiber foods like beans, bananas, raspberries, collard greens, broccoli, and live culture bacteria for regular maintenance.

Seaweed

Also known as a sea vegetable and macroalgae contains fiber, antioxidants and numerous vitamins and minerals. Rich in iron, calcium, magnesium and manganese, and iodine. Anyone who suffers from Thyroid problems and need a rich antioxidant, vitamins and minerals would benefit from this sea vegetable. Consuming this throughout the day daily is a bonus!

Magnesium

Regulates blood sugar and reduces the risk of diabetes. Stimulating brain growth, magnesium was the first to play a major role in alleviating depression and anxiety. Food source is leafy green, seeds, avocado, legumes, bananas, vegetables like greens, kale, and spinach. A serving of greens contains almost .16 grams of magnesium.

Phytonutrients

Phytonutrients help decrease the risk of many illnesses of cancer threat and disease. Considered thousands of nutrients and oxygen are found in plants to support the cells in our body from disease. Found in red fruits, orange, and vegetables.

Greens, cabbage, broccoli, cauliflower, Brussel sprouts, spinach, avocado, spinach, cucumber, ginger, turmeric, purple onions are popular to lower blood pressure, improve heart, deliver high potent immunity, and render digestion issues. All of them are high in vitamin and render therapeutic cell recovery in the body. Bananas in my opinion were the best at providing a fiber and high antioxidant, worthier identical to a ginger or turmeric shot drink supplement to boost immunity. I would sometimes go to a local upscale grocery to grab a ginger shot or turmeric supplement drink. I would also grab a all organic gingerade live culture drink for drinking on an empty stomach to detox the gut.

Detoxing on an empty stomach just accelerates the absorption of antioxidants. Other times I would buy a ginger drink with lemon or a chlorophyll aloe organic mixture. Each day, all consumed on an empty stomach for maximum effect. The same as taking a prescription on an empty stomach. Then followed with an antioxidant alkaline vegetable meal or snack. When I say snack, I mean seeds, nuts, berries, sliced fruit, seaweed, or broth soup with mushrooms. Leaving plenty of room for the main course alkaline meal. Use caution when cooking vegetables for mold, or how to cook it without deep frying with vegetable and canola oil. Essentially, cooking it in the most-healthiest way, which is steamed, boiled or sir fry with olive oil and antioxidant seasons. Depending on the specific taste bud, will depend on what is prepared. For all beans organically, must be soaked for a couple of hours. So be mindful in the preparation of cooking up alkaline vegetables in a timely manner by having certain vegetables prepped.

Day to day, contents of antioxidants and the delivery of nutrients throughout the digestive system in the morning is almost like a shot of whiskey or identical to the social dependency puffing of a cigarette or cigar. Coincidently, I had always craved green tea before knowing the benefits of its' purpose. Starting off with green tea was a seamless transition. Green tea contains high amounts of catechins, which are antioxidants suggested to help prevent cell damage and it's considered one of the world's healthiest most popular teas. A detox drink combining 3 small fresh slices of organic ginger (high powerful antioxidant), maybe add a mint, 3 squirts of lemon juice or 3 slices (for cleansing the gastro lining of the digestive system), three spoons of apple cider vinegar (kills bacteria) and 3 medium shots of organic honey for natural sweetness. Detoxing was the end of smoking, drinking alcohol, and eating saturated fat for me. Essentially, because it would defeat the purpose of starting a new conferment to ending it. It's like letting out bad people in jail who was taken off the streets for murder and putting them back out on the street to do it again. Quitting smoking and drinking my detox made my throat go from a hot exhaust pipe of a car that had been continuously running from California to New York, to an iced lake. Its' like I could feel the rendered smoothness of a fresh start. Smiling to myself when hearing the transition of my voice getting lighter and healthier from drinking this antioxidant. So, you can just about imagine how this became a therapeutic antioxidant smoothness for me. Along with the high potency of fresh ginger and other high antioxidants, clearing up my bronchi, liver, and kidneys, down throughout my digestive system. Notice, I left out the reproductive system because this muscle is targeted the most with healthier immunity and blood circulation as it's best prevention. Despite there is no researched test of this, eating healthy will always filter good circulation health. Again, though some disorders are uncontrollable, blood transports healthy enzymes to revive new formulated cells for better organ health.

Note: Quitting cigarettes is often unbreakable, so it may require plenty of fresh cut lemon in water or lemon juice on the tongue to aid in flushing the toxic addictions out the body.

Merely trademark, this process of drinking green tea to detox the digestive system. The reason I say this is, not only was this the beginning of flushing out toxins and keeping me regular with high antioxidants, but this is also my ritual. I had to keep mind this was a consistent clearing and shedding of toxic dead/damage cells, removing pathogen in organs, and toning my skin. Again, some people have no choice but to be on medication. However, don't let it stop you from eating this way.

Granted I'm aware that if my body can no longer fight the damages, my next step would be to go to a licensed physician. I am not a God and sometimes a physician can quickly tell you if things are or may not be on the right path. Which is why I had to take this route at first, instead of being uninformed or getting bounced around in the healthcare system. When I can apply the same costs of prescription medication to eating a straight alkaline antioxidant diet. Or later end up on all kinds of medication or short lived going to see different physicians due to side effect issues from previous prescribed medication. Its' hard to imagine if I had not been consuming alkaline foods as a remedy to live a healthier less complicated and excessive visits to the doctor what would I be doing. Would I be broke, or barely working going back and forth to the Dr.? Or am I going to spend my time eating everything natural for longevity? You see, why would anyone want to think about a bad dream when you know it's a bad dream, so undermine it control your own destiny.

As a primary premise for drinking this to cleanse my digestive tract, my digestive tract can start rebuilding new healthy cellular function inside my intestinal walls. Yes, the same walls that polyps form in the digestive tract that can sometimes ignite into colon cancer. At which can be exaggerated by either abuse to the body (bad food, cigarette, alcohol) or from inheritance. This abuse does damage to the cilia within the intestine which is responsible for censoring chemical changes in the contents of molecules in the bowel. Destroying this must be repaired to prevent buildup of dead, damaged, or unneeded cellular growth in the body. You must remember, the digestive tract is responsible for transferring nutrients to the cells for repair and growth to include the skin. So, when it comes to toxicity, it slowly damages the skin, the stomach, then spreading throughout the entirety of the digestive system. Affecting other organs like the reproductive system, liver, kidneys, all other organs properties.

The digestive tract essentially, has a major purpose to share the wealth to all parts of the body to include the brain. Just think to yourself when taking a prescription via mouth, it must go through the stomach and digestive system for it to work. Which sometimes is a waiting process. So, you can get my point when drinking this mixture of green tea and antioxidant ingredients in the morning on an empty stomach will do for the stomach, digestive system, and overall body. Throughout the time it takes for your body to breakdown consuming alkaline foods, your system is in constant reconstruction of antioxidant behavior. Instead of damaging your organs to break down unhealthy acidic foods. If your, not a green tea drinker I would suggest experimenting with drinking another organic antioxidant tea with the same high antioxidant ingredients that I previously mentioned. It is mandatory to replace drinking coffee to green tea or another detox in the morning. Even when the ingredients to coffee are not present, it is still a non-antioxidant.

If you have constipation issues like irritable bowel syndrome, I once suffered as a continuous side effect while taking medication for back pain before starting this alkaline lifestyle of course, adding a teaspoon of castor oil also does wonders for the digestive tract. Castor oil used as a laxative that can help fight constipation, however it cannot be used long-term because it is a laxative. A laxative can cause other issues to occur if abused.

It's top reality as we get to 35 our weight gain is faster, and our energy is desensitized. So, to keep consistent and divert from slowing down I would continue eating seeds and antioxidant snacks in between the afternoon and evening hours. Mainly I would bring alkaline snacks (nuts, seeds, dates, seeded crackers, seaweed, or alkaline fruit) throughout the day to prevent me from hunger or relapsing. Relapsing temptation that could send me back to eating unhealthy cheap fast-food snacks like fries or fried food. With the help of deploying abstinence from processed foods and animal meat my intake of antioxidant alkaline food and snacks contributed to no weight gain. Because meat and processed foods take longer to digest it sits longer in our intestines, I consumed either o or hardly any calories. Not to mention, I wasn't entertaining saturated fat. As a matter of facts, fecal mass stuck in the colon can lead to illness or even death. Whereas alkaline releases natural energy enzymes that don't take the body to long to absorb and digest toxin. Leaving me to feel expunged and bloat free from damageable waste in my gut. I was able to assume eating unhealthy big or excessive meals caused me to be sleepy, constipated, gassy, bloated, and overall sluggish. Whereas eating alkaline antioxidant gave me energy, a naturally cleaner gut, and organs.

When eating peanuts, walnuts, bitter apricots, healthy nuts and apples or fruit with an organic antioxidant drink to change things up I would bring a bowel of beans and rice and a fruit and drink. Beans like white beans are high in iron, kidney beans are essentially good for the kidneys, chic-peas help remove harmful radicals and black beans are rich in antioxidants. Keep in mind organic beans must soaked in water for about 2 hours before cooking.

Since the rise of plant-based foods, the richer antioxidants are beginning to become affordably priced for their function in upscale supermarkets. Casually, this is what I did to diversify eating to keep steady throughout the day.

Reiterating on the topic of the parasympathetic nervous system, when your brain must switch its focus to digest the food that is needed to aid the body's immunity, the unhealthier the harder it puts pressure and exertion on your organs. You see, the brain must operate the micro-organisms response to the body's immunity. This part of the brain is called the insula. The insula is the superior control tower over the parasympathetic nervous system to the stomach. Gastro functions are changed, if evoked, if increased parasympathetic plunge occurs. When I consumed alkaline foods every day consistently no eating meat, I stabilized healthy weight-loss, brain function, throughout the day, for a healthier immune system. Outlining my evening with my schedule of days' I jogged for thirty minutes', best in the early a.m.'s is mainly when I could afford to do cardio. If not, I would have to alter it to the evening. Closely making sure I didn't devour a big alkaline meal or increase stomach fullness before running in the evening.

Cardio daily was a top priority to detox saturated fat under my skin, in my muscles, organs in my body. Anything my body didn't need which was unwarranted fat and unstable cells, bringing down the physics of my immunity. Contrary to unwarranted fat, the body does need healthy fat to use to absorb the nutrients and vitamins like A, D, and E. In which, vitamin E is most important because it serves as a function to protect cells from free radical damage. These healthy fats are called polyunsaturated and monounsaturated fat. Essentially polyunsaturated and monounsaturated fats is a good healthy fat soluble for the body, uses for good energy and aide for vitamins and minerals to be absorbed. So, instead of saturated oil, skillet alkaline vegetable with avocado or olive oil because they are polyunsaturated and monosaturated.

Seafood boiled, steamed, or grilled is also an alkaline property. It is low in calorie when steamed, boiled, or grilled. <u>Seafood is also a rich protein non-acidic and does not contain saturated fat</u>. If it is not cooked with butter, vegetable, canola oil or deeply fried. Another equivalent to eating polyunsaturated and monounsaturated fat would be avocado, beans, rice, brown noodles and even tofu. Before I became routine to this miracle diet, I would fast throughout the day mostly, then eat a big meal of an alkaline antioxidant light olive or avocado oil skillet entrée for dinner and get sleepy immediately. I would sometime just focus on emptying out my body that every time I wanted to eat something, I became more conscious of what was in it and what could harm my body. I would eat mainly boiled or steamed alkaline organic veggies (not in a can) with brown or white rice and rich organic antioxidant beans so much that I was thankful more plant-based foods hit the market. Six years living on an alkaline lifestyle, is when I finally incorporated boiled, steamed, or grilled seafood unsaturated with certain dinners of skillet alkaline vegetables. Sometimes, during the day after a year of this alkaline diet, I would eat sushi for lunch, without all the cream cheese and additives of course. With a broth or sometimes a seafood broth. I didn't want to slow down my metabolism and make my body sleepy most days, so this would be random. At rest the body is essential to muscle growth. So, for instance, when you exercise, the muscles rip, at rest the muscles, called fibroblasts repair. The parasympathetic system is responsible for when the body is a rest. For example, when breathing slowly with deep breaths can trigger the parasympathetic nervous system. The parasympathetic nervous system initiates the muscles in the digestive system for relaxation of the muscles to occur. Lowering our blood pressure at the same time, especially after a stressful situation. Relaxation breeds recovery in the body. Have you ever heard of an old tale that saying you grow in your sleep? Truth behold that is what sleeping does for my body, recovering my muscles and my body. Contrary to the parasympathetic nervous system is the sympathetic nervous system. Which is the division of the body's energy response. The sympathetic nervous system when acceleration occurs dilates bronchioles circulating with adrenaline. Say for instance you have a cold, the bronchioles become inflamed. When you exercise the bronchioles dilate, which is important to help us breath better, especially when we have a cold. Perspiration is the exchange of heat respiration in the body. When eating energy like alkaline green leafy vegetables that contain many nutrients like Vitamin A, B-complex, calcium, magnesium, and iron, this initiates the sympathetic nervous system. Leaning to fasting or snacking on alkaline snacks during the day stimulate the body's flight or fight response as much as possible to keep energy of antioxidants flowing.

Alkaline fruits are filled with antioxidant structed seeds of a plant. You can agree or disagree that seeds are bountiful and extremely nutritious for the major parts of the body. Few can be harmful to our gastro-intestinal disturbances. Yet majority, they are high antioxidant and protein seeds for the organs in the body. They have a good source of minerals, B, E, and selenium vitamins. Selenium boosts your immune system, reduces our age decline, reducing the effects of heart disease and some forms of cancer. However, consuming over 400 mcg reportedly is an unsafe dose. On the flip side, imagine eating a cup of mixed pecans, chestnuts, peanuts, pistachios, and sunflower seeds for a total antioxidant richness. All are high potent little pellets. And considered a useful hunger crave ammunition. Poppy seeds, bitter apricot, cashew nuts, flax seeds, sesame seeds, almonds, Brazil nuts, and chia seeds are all high antioxidant seeds. Chia seeds has shown to reduce blood sugar immediately after a meal. Overall, chia seeds contain several antioxidant polyphenols. In conclusion, alkaline seeds are an effective essential antioxidant property. Intake of only these seeds every day maximized my immune system to an alkaline environment.

Depending on your taste for certain fruits, here is a list of alkaline fruits to plan and perhaps even mix the vegetables together in a water cup, fruit bowl or blended into a smoothie:

Blackberries

Berries

Cherries

Strawberries

Green or Red Apples,

Banana

Cantaloupe

Melon

Watermelon

Figs, Raisins, Dates

Pears, Peaches

Tangerine

Oranges

Mango

Kiwi

Papaya

Grapefruit

Grapes

Apricots

Plums

Pineapple

Aloe plant

Eating seeds intermittently to prevent hunger in between the hours of the day also kept me energized. I also would make an organic gluten free whole grain oatmeal on some days just that just to circulate nothing, but the entirety of every vitamin absorbed. Or an avocado, tomato and cucumber sandwich with sesame and black seeds all day or eat two a day along with antioxidant alkaline water. Essentially building an internal wall of antioxidants. Avoiding interaction with anyone or eating around unhealthy eating. Without a firm non-negotiable mental perception, reverting to unhealthy foods just minimizes prevention. Again, overtime once the body gets used to not eating a big plate of unhealthy food, it will readjust the control of hunger and use up healthy fat at a consistent velocity. Using my mind to pass over tempting to eat an unhealthy meal or snack. For many of years, the practice of fasting, which is to abstain from food for specific periods of the day or time has been a popular concept of ridding the body from impurities. Fasting reduces inflammation allows cells to repair and improves overall fitness. Your body autonomously loses up to 50 calories during fasting.

Wheat is not necessarily organic because it is combined with other ingredients like flour and baked. However, it is still an essential antioxidant if it is organic gluten free, with maybe flax, sesame, or chia seeds added on top, as a better choice of fiber and protein than white bread. So, if you are like me, and want to still stop at your favorite coffee shop, a wheat bagel that contains flax seeds, sesame, black or chia seeds is a healthy antioxidant and natural healthy alkaline on the go fat burner (polyunsaturated fat). I've even seen some organic juice shops that have opened along my journey that offer alkaline fruit in a blended smoothie no sugar or organic honey of course. For example, I like getting a green apple, blended kale, and kiwi drink with ginger and honey on the go. If there's a chance to buy vegan crackers or wheat chips, it will also be one of my favorite combination with cucumbers and almond butter. Just ensure you look at the ingredients on the nutrition label to ensure it does not contain high acidity or saturated/trans-fat higher than 2% if nothing else it is organic without GMO ingredients and preservatives. Even if it has a little sprinkle of salt make sure its sea salt or a low percentage. Casually still drink plenty of lemon/apple cider vinegar and cucumber water. Today, there are many vegan appetizers in restaurants and snacks for on the go, in gas stations or grocery stores. Any person can access an alkaline food only diet on the go conveniently.

It's all about knowing what is alkaline and what contains rich antioxidants to expedite oxidation and healing to be restored. Vegan entrées are so popularized, that now it's going to lead into a drive-through. Particularly in larger cities first. Which further confirms that a plant- based lifestyle is unquestionably growing a public trust. Especially, as health care expenses and illness rise all around the world, many are using this as a safer way to live. So, next time remind yourself why eating vegetarian is popular. Eliminating animal processed foods will only help the body stay free from acidic animal fat, inflamed blood, or other diseases from what the animals eat.

Furthermore, adding to research, since an alkaline environment reduces the dangers of inflammation in the body, a common illness such as sinusitis (which is blockage of the sinus cavity from a cold or allergy) will experience no triggers from intolerance from alkaline food. Damage from inflammation evaporates initially. It's no questions an alkaline diet increases the body's immunity to speed off the fight against a virus, even at rest does more than speed up the fight against the virus.

GETTING STARTED

Consider for once that you have a meal designed to carry on the go, at work and, during work for 7 days?

You'll agree with me that it gets easier when you can look at a one-day meal plan at a time. Surrounded with snacks of antioxidants. This is the importance of a learned behavior – one that taught me how to remain consistent without expending much time in how and what to prepare. Just becoming mentally trained was the hard part. But once I got to the top, regular eating became consistent.

When I began the alkaline kickoff, and my fate to keep my body non-acidic, if I had to recreate a visual of the meal journey, I would begin at the first day of the week, (Sunday) as the best way to get a conversant schedule physical transparency. What I mean by this is, knowing how to prepare foods, quickly and having fresh fruits and seeds on hand. Basically, knowing what I was going to already make and which way I was going to prepare it. Using Saturday, as my prep day for getting utensils, storage, and inventory together. Ultimately, prepared to not look back. For over a decade now, I can honestly say that not every day in the morning I drink green hot tea with added detox ingredients that I mentioned before. The reason for this is because sometimes my body can get tired of the same detox edible. Alternate drinking a detox in the morning with fasting with a ginger organic shot drink, or organic turmeric shot. Other times an organic pineapple, turmeric and orange combined high in vitamin C probiotic drink or an algae chlorophyll drink to offset overindulgence of green tea. Drinking chlorophyll helped regulate cholesterol, digestion and neutralize toxins. If I didn't already eat an alkaline meal for the day, I would consume this on an empty stomach. Doing this allowed me to feel it go down my esophagus and stomach. Having complete control over rejuvenating my body with only antioxidants.

A creative alkaline combination of rice and black beans in a small bowl with cucumber or avocado is a petite size that I consumed throughout the workday, mainly because it was easy to warm up in a container. Not to eat too much but in-between I would eat snacks of nuts, organic fruit, or seeded wheat crackers. No candy, no chocolate, no coffee, no sugar, and no soda. No cigarettes either. Just antioxidant organic unpasteurized food.

If I perceived I was not able to boil rice or have time for organic beans, I would make a bowl or salad of romaine or spring lettuce with a mixture of baby spinach and broccoli, mushrooms. With sometimes a sliced purple cabbage, purple onion, tomatoes, sunflower seeds or raisins or dried natural fruit berries topped with olive oil and apple cider vinegar is what I opt for as an edible condiment. Yes, the concept of trying different salads and snacks with alkaline vegetables helps curb the thoughts of reverting back to carbs, meat, and extra fat foods. Besides that, experimenting with different organic rice and beans is a good base to be topped with skillet or steamed vegetables. I can admit after so many years of only eating this way, I began making steamed or boiled seafood on the side. Generally, 4 times a month. Other than that, I would venture to an upscale grocery markets to find more organic snacks that are non-acidic and plentiful of antioxidants. They didn't contain preservatives or that food that contains high fructose syrup, artificial flavors, GMO, and extra sweeteners.

Eating broccoli salad with sunflower, pumpkin seeds or your choice, red onions, and sweet peas or chickpeas also serves as a delicious salad. I can't stress enough to shuffle alkaline vegetables into big and little creations, as much as possible. Some salads can be simply made with peas or chickpeas, cucumbers, olives, kidney beans with steamed mushroom and broccoli. Recommended with a vegan salad dressing or avocado, almond, olive oil with apple cider vinegar, olives, oregano, and sea salt as seasoning. Sometimes I get creative and add garlic or turmeric powder and cayenne pepper. Cayenne pepper is a detox agent for weight-loss, boosts metabolism with anti- inflammatory properties. Cayenne pepper also has a high source of provitamin A and vitamin C. Garlic powder is combined with antioxidants and minerals that aid in the support of the immune system. Working as a siren to warn off flu and bacterial infections.

Heavy drinking lots of natural organic ingredient water with sliced fruit drinks, organic broth, organic vegetable juice or two bottles of water for flushing my liver. Flushing out viruses, cysts coagulation and dead or unwanted cellular growth. Probiotic bacteria organic drinks that are non-acidic a good culture of bacteria that kept my gut hydrated and back in to balance throughout the day. Pineapple with apple, celery, probiotic Bifidobacterium, saccharomyces and Lactobacillus and orange drink all day does great improvement for the digestive system. Remember to be consistent to clean up anything and everything of concern.

In the winter, its' imperative to keep the body filled with organic broth soup to balance the body's temperature. My most recommended broth consumption is one in which I would add a spring of lemon juice and a little of apple cider vinegar - primarily because it has the immense ability to clean the colon and detoxing the mucous membranes descending from the throat through the intestines. If you are unaware of the anti-inflammatory benefits of lemon and limes, you will find that it is an essential antioxidant and detox agent to add to broth and salads. Even boiling organic beans can benefit an extra bonus with lemon or lime. I absolutely eliminated drinking soda or diet soda of any kind. Again, the results show. Hence, daily drinking of lemon juice and water is a high detox compound agent that not only works well, as you know for the digestive system, aids to help reduce acne breakouts by decreasing inflammation also. Some people I came across would drink this with sliced cucumbers as well. Keep in mind lemon juice is acidic but once it's digested it does many wonders for the bodies' immune health and to the intestine by loosening the toxins in the GI tract. So, I didn't worry much about the use of lemon slices or juice in almost every meal during the alignment of my internal environment to be more alkaline since this is detoxing my system. Sometimes, I would boil water, and cut lemon and cucumber and pour together in a pitcher and put it in the refrigerator to drink throughout the week.

As you may have figured, dinner is not the same anymore. No more three course meals with a meat. Just for it to travel around the body and negatively affect my weight and organs. I read a particular column once and it said the Western diet tends to eat a full meal until we are full, presupposing that it was the dominant factor responsible for an obese culture. Then what happens after we eat a full meal; we get sleepy and then food gets stored in the organs (visceral fat). Not forgetting to mention, how long it takes to digest through the digestive system. And what I was getting in return. After comparing the results from my past weight gain to a now detoxed body, I can see that neither my body nor my colon needed a full unhealthy stool. For instance, fast food fried meals, because this is the many of reasons that cause weight gain, contributed to my Graves' disease diagnosis. Hyper activating my hormones secretions into a negative side effect.

Eating animal and processed meat or bio engineered ingredients did the opposite of eating alkaline food to my Grave's disease. Only reducing inflammation and loading it with an insulin production of antioxidant cellular function. On days I felt unoccupied, I would dip into a fast-food restaurant to eat something quickly. I would have no choice but to have a side salad, even though it is rumored that not all salad is organic, this was the only time I would take a chance. At other locations I would buy side vegetables items like red beans and rice or cooked greens. But today, its' even easier to order an alkaline meal for about 15.00 or less at certain foreign or small restaurants. Indian and Philippine restaurants are known for their organic alkaline no meat entrees. Or a vegetarian restaurant depending on where you live. Other than that, the most cost-effective way is cooking at home. I can't argue that it's dreadful lust to smell those French fries and burgers, or fried chicken when out traveling. I somehow overtime, have built a trust and conscience with myself when I smell it lingering in the air, whether I'm outdoors or indoors somewhere, that its' not healthy. Remembering what's in the contents, its' origin and history. Single handedly would I think about all the food I would like to eat before leaving this world, but then I remind myself, it wouldn't matter what I didn't eat when I'm not living. So, while I'm here it is my prayer to remain consistent in eating alkaline antioxidants to help continuously fight the internal issues inside my body to live a longer fight.

DAILY MODERATION

Sunday, I started off drinking green tea of course, with antioxidant vegetable agents like organic ginger root sliced, sliced lemons, 3 spoons of apple cider vinegar and organic honey in the morning. I transition lunch into a recommended two servings of hot broth with mushrooms and celery apple cider vinegar or lemon juice (Japanese clear soup). Even on the go I would bring it in a coffee-like drinking cup. To dry out mucous from the nasal, throat, and chest cavity. Added to lunch if no time for snacks, I either take natural mashed potatoes with broccoli or mix into a broth soup sliced individually. And sometimes I make a blackeye peas with brown rice, or green lima beans with quinoa rice (gluten-free) on the side of the soup or in replace. Depending on how I am feeling. Sometimes an avocado or asparagus, a complementing compound of a solid intake of antioxidants for lunch, but without large consumption to prevent major rest & digest.

Monday

Monday is the normal reasonable top of the day in a work week for some. The mindset I repeated in my head was that I am always removing the toxic tumor cells and harmful agents from my body. The first thing I think of when I'm waking up getting my day started. Implementing the expectation and motivation to see and feel results with each day in the end not wanting to feel regrets. I wouldn't consume eggs because they came from chicken. There are vegan eggs, however, I haven't tried them still to this day. I hear they are plant-based eggs. Regular eggs are the same as eating meat so to speak. So, if you are wanting to detox your body from acid, forget about eggs in the morning, unless it is vegan eggs. Eggs are acid-forming and although it is high in protein it has a moderate level of 6.0 to 6.5 and that's soft, cooked. I would buy my son cage free eggs boil or scramble white yolk, because I trusted it to be healthier than eating eggs that are in overpopulated housing. For weight loss concerns yolk from eggs is considered to have high cholesterol. However, I still did not consume eggs. Since alkaline consists of keeping the bodies pH to 7.0, one egg is acidic enough. So, what I would do is rotate my alkaline choices for one breakfast nutrient with another which I listed in previous reference. I would rotate my favorites to my least favorite depending on the day of the week and work schedule to reduce hungriness' and continue my high intake of alkaline in the morning.

Depending on how stretched a person's tummy is, may also depend on how much nutrients to supply the body with. Meaning, if I'm at work, the best thing to do is keep a cult of organic snack whole or sliced fruit in a bag and nuts on the side. For record, my skin began to glow from after 3 days of detox, and my body's digestive system well you know, I went on days and years forgetting about the symptomatic complaints I use to have i.e., constipation or IBS, Graves' Disease flair-ups. From the appearance of my skin, I was able to see the difference in comparison up close in a person faces if he or she consumes processed foods versus an alkaline antioxidant diet consumed daily in moderation. The appearance of healthy ageless skin versus someone who is not is transparent enough. The obvious is mistaken for compliments of "you look younger", but your thoughts are reckoning with your doubts of this becoming a life-long transition lifestyle because of the visibility of detoxed skin internally.

Some may argue that it doesn't matter how healthy you eat, we still die. Which is true, but if your able to out-live your doubts about uncontrollable health problems, keeping your digest intact with alkaline food you can reinvent organ function. Over time compressing the loss of your bone strength and joint mobility to get around better. Dreading as we age with lesser pain and grace. Nonetheless, constant prescription medication for inflammation or the onset-of disease as we age can cause side effects. Making it harder on organs to operate normal activities like getting out the bed without nausea. Common causes of nausea are brought on by antibiotics, opioids, anti-depressants, and medicines used to treat cancer. Other causes of nausea are emotional stress, gall bladder disease, food poisoning, or infections. Although, there are diseases that cannot be avoided for instance, hereditary diseases, that is incurable, in most cases where nothing can be done. Yet still, the body stands a better chance of fighting inflammation in an alkaline environment.

Tuesday

As the journey follows my newness to strive, Tuesday, I continue thinking of rotating my green tea. To a tall glass of almond milk by itself or blended with strawberry, kiwi, and bananas. Or an organic orange juice with strawberries. Or organic apple juice with aloe plant and pineapples. Organic prune juice, or if possible, blend your own vegetable high antioxidant combination of a vegetable and fruit. The reason for organic drinks is to eliminate pesticides and any preservatives used to make it last longer. It also contains less pollution. Preservatives can weaken the hearts tissue. Sometimes they contain cancer causing additives as well as disrupting our hormones. Disabling the objective of the hormones ability to be effective. When I was restricted to liquids, these drinks were the only drinks that would fill me up with antioxidants and nutrients. For lunch, sometimes I would drink two ensures (vanilla protein as my preference). In the winter, I would mainly consume one or two cups of warmed tomato soup on-the-go (grocery organic soup), broth or mushroom soup. Broth kicks off a flavor packed with vitamin, folate, calcium, and magnesium. Keeping the immune system fighting infection with extra hydration. For 6 weeks, I continued to go to school during my jaw injury reconstruction, as I mentioned before I had liquids only. So, the potency of drinking lots of natural organic juices does reduce hungriness throughout my day. It can be done to live drinking antioxidants, vitamins, and minerals.

Wednesday

Wednesday is that hump in the middle of the week, that always seems to endow as an overseer of delay. You can think of it as a midway mission accomplished milestone. What I mean by that is, I use this day to orchestrate combining other alkaline fruits & vegetables based on taste bud and budget ability. Meaning it's easy for someone to suggest a meal, but in my journey, it works better with the person's preference's on trying different alkaline foods that entice you to eat more or combine creativeness. Mixing different antioxidant seasoning with organic flavoring. There's no real book on preparing meals that are alkaline. It's simply steamed alkaline or boiled vegetables with organic brown rice or brown noodles with high intakes of antioxidant fruits and vegetables. They can either be sliced and ate on the side or scrambled. For example, I would slice cucumbers and avocado to go on top or on the side with brown rice chickpeas and spinach.

When making organic beans, they must be soaked for 2 hours before cooking. I would still add apple cider vinegar and lemon juice to my beans to prepare. Even when I skillet some cabbage broccoli, onions, and mushrooms, I would put 4 tablespoons of olive oil, teaspoon of ginger turmeric, apple cider vinegar and cayenne pepper. Then put the vegetables on top of the seasoning. Even though its' Wednesday, detox of green tea is still what I needed to filter through my intestine to attack any bad buildup. You can switch your blend, but apple cider vinegar is important for detoxing even the colon. Apple cider contains agents responsible when ingested to excrete agents of bad bacteria, toxin, and dead cells out the body. Even in the grocery store, you may have seen an apple cider vinegar water mix drink for digestive system detoxing. After flushing with the consumption of apple cider vinegar, I would eat a banana or have something probiotic organic for my gut an hour later. And drink this on the go, until lunch. Coating my colon with rich antioxidant, good bacteria, potassium, and vitamin C. Potassium helps improve the nerves in the heart to contract regularly along with helping nutrients move into cells and waste out of cells.

Referencing bananas, with high amounts of potassium, it also is a healthy fiber that aids in weight loss. Fiber is the process of pushing food through your body without dissolving in water. Essentially, aiding in removing waste from the digestive system and thus lowering cholesterol levels. Another occupation to add about eating banana's is that it also fights inflammation in the joints for arthritis and inflammation. Still keep in mind this worked effectively for me without all the preservatives, artificial, bio-engineered and meat interferences. I would consume a banana at least 3 or 4 times a week. Which I struggled to remember to do consistently after months of this lifestyle. So, unless you are disciplined in wanting the best chance of recovery, create a schedule or reminders of what to eat. Almost identical to a pill separator, you know what color and quantity to take at a certain time of the day. Note: too much fiber without plenty of water (detoxing with lemon/lime/ or cucumber water) can cause constipation. Attempting too much of one fruit or specific vegetable only detached me from the desire of eating it at all reason being my mind would draw a blank on what to eat next. However, I still would eat a bowl of strawberries, berries, apples, and cucumber at least 4 times a week. Or sometimes I would switch it around to withstand from repetitive behavior. I'm sure that can happen to anyone, if you eat pizza everyday soon or later the brain tells you that your tired of eating pizza, so you must jog your memory on something else you like to eat, or I would fast. Wednesday is the tip of the week, you must change gears, relax more and fast to accomplish more meals for the rest of the week to come. Your able to grasp the openness to your objectives and reflect on what you can improve next.

\When I would catch a cold (virus) that mainly caused me to have symptoms of congestion, cough, to fever all from the inflammation of a virus attacking my healthy immune system. When this would happen before being on an alkaline diet my symptoms were way worse, and I needed medication to relieve symptoms. On an alkaline diet, my symptoms weren't severe to require over the counter medication or antibiotic prescription medication for symptoms of a virus. I would consume more amounts of fresh ginger root with sliced lemon or lime with green tea and apple cider vinegar to intake. The ginger internally attacked the mucous congestion in my nasal cavity down to my chest. Once you taste an organic ginger, you will taste the same flavor in modern cough medicine.

Historically, there was criticism of holistic natural eating. Eating a plant-based alkaline lifestyle is what our ancestor survived hundreds of years consuming to renovate the body from disease forming radicals. The other popular criticism is eating meat. Without eating meat that it's said that you deprive your body from protein, muscle and thus cannot survive without meat. Which is stereotypical if you ask me. Coming from a person who refused to take stool softeners, hormone, and inflammatory medication to control my Grave's Disease, I have better results in my digestive system, hormones, and skin from cutting out meat and eating alkaline foods. I also replaced eating meat with a natural protein from Tofu (which can be marinated seasoned grilled for sandwich or pasta bowl). I generally after constant drinking of skillet combined alkaline foods, would I incorporate tofu as a supplement for meat as a sandwich or I would buy vegetarian sandwich meat in an upscale grocery market to eat as well. I know what you are thinking, have I ever reverted to eating anything else. Answer is yes, I realized as I mentioned before, that many of our seafood friends contain high antioxidants and protein. So, one thing that did not disrupt my alkaline balance was grilled shrimp with olive oil or avocado oil or steamed shrimp. I would stay away from butter, vegetable, canola oil all together. Vegetable and canola oil are saturated fats, that settle in the front of your belly. In which will also travel around the body. Essentially, depositing specks of fat, lining around the organs making it harder to burn stomach fat. A supporting evident to my remark is the infamous belly tea drinks that allegedly burn belly fat. Just flip to the ingredients and see what agents are inside the contents of a tummy fat burner. I researched on this intervention, the ingredients contain apple cider vinegar and green tea along with other weight loss leaves.

The biggest mental deflection when first adapting to only alkaline food is the craving for fast food or unhealthy snacks like chips, chocolate, which only happens when we experience fast hunger relief. An occurrence when I sat there and calculated how long of a sequence does it ache and what stretching I can do to disrupt it, didn't require a meal. May sound dangerous to you but think for a moment what did humans eat on the go 400 years ago? How often they may have fasted. There are natural sweeteners like pomegranate, mangos, strawberries, berries, watermelons, and melons to snack on for sweet delight. Along with adding pineapples and kiwi. All that can be blended as an organic fruit delighted drink to have as a slushy or cold beverage. In all it supplies the sweet cravings we get from time to time. Again, scheduling what to cook will you be able to achieve the week and so on further as a lifestyle. It is identical to the concept of eating different fast food at different places you know you have the weekly budget for.

On times I'd bring a bowl or sandwich bag of apples, grapes and nuts or seeds, would the apples promote fullness and reduce the appetite to eat. Apples contain a flavonoid which is essential to lower the chances of heart disease, blood pressure and acting as an antioxidant just so you know. Simultaneously, grapes are high in potassium vitamins, minerals and is associated to the prevention of cancer. Let's not forget to have at least 2 water bottles or drink that is organic. Again, it can be something of a water organic honey drink mixed with berries, strawberries, cucumbers, and lemon. The fuller you are from organic alkaline foods and juice or water the less stress of being hunger, the more alkaline the internal environment is. Celery sticks with an almond butter and a healthy quick cabbage wrap is a great alkaline food snack. You may have seen those clear wraps that look like it's a bunch of veggies in it like a taco. Brewing organic broth soup with maybe fresh mushrooms and green onions with a simple salad of fresh green leaves was also another favorite alkaline put together assortment. You can even add shrimp, fresh salmon, or tofu to help control the crave for meat, but keep in mind 80 % plant 20 % seafood or Tofu.

Continue alternating alkaline seeded snacks to have fun with your life.

When on the way home eating a mixture of alkaline snacks like perhaps raisins, dates (acts as a brain booster, reducing blood sugar and blood pressure antioxidant), almond, walnuts or sprouted crackers with tangerine or watermelon gives you time to take your mind from rushing home to cook dinner or feeling exhausted. Because again, emptying the stomach from processed, greasy, genetically modified food, it will feel different to eat less and feel less hunger. It's almost as if I had to starve the body from toxic acidic genetically modified fast food to alkaline food to eliminate the toxins level created to trick the body into fullness because it takes longer to digest.

Dinner would include a quinoa rice, sliced avocado on the side with (olive, coconut, or olive oil) skillet with alkaline veggies, sprouts, potatoes, broccoli, cauliflower, zucchini, cucumber, sliced tomato, and some sort of vegan spread of choice, veggie broth soup with baked or grilled tofu sort of arrangement. Seasoned with garlic, turmeric, cayenne pepper, sea salt and oregano. Remember this is an exclusion of processed man-made foods, so I typically bought as many green filled vegetables as possible and added baby spinach to my broth with apple cider vinegar and lemon. And just simply put things together like bean sprouts, celery, mushrooms, and brown noodles I remember seeing at a Thai, Philippine, or Indian restaurant.

Note: Sometimes I would leave a bowl of blackeye peas soaking in water on the counter for two hours in the morning. Then when I would arrive home to later boil with apple cider vinegar to eat with brown or quinoa rice, onions, green peppers, and mushrooms. This would take about 2 hours to boil after soaking for two hours. This is when I would say a crockpot is going to come in handy. Another very delicious alkaline meal is chic-peas with quinoa rice, topped with onions, peppers, mushrooms and alkaline seasoning. Quinoa is packed with anti-inflammatory phytonutrients that aid the body with higher benefits in the prevention of disease. If I had not soaked my beans, it would have taken way more time to cook.

The importance of eating grown organic beans and vegetables is because canned and frozen vegetables can deplete their nutritional value.

In the morning have a green blended smoothie; ingredient can include but not all (green apple, kale, cut cucumbers, organic honey, ginger root, and ice). Again, giving the body a citrus of alkalinity in the morning.

Take with you another couple of fruit of choice with bottles of water. I know many people who literally slice in half an avocado, remove the seed, and essentially eat the avocado with a spoon. I do this as well, however, I add salt and pepper, cayenne, and turmeric on both sides to add a tang to it.

Thursday is a bit simpler. Drinking simply two on-the-go tomato, mushroom, cream of broccoli soup or celery soup that can be warmed up in a microwave. Or simply an ensure. Depending on the craving to eat add celery sticks and almond butter for snack. Or perhaps cut apples and berries. Black, blue and raspberries contain the highest antioxidants in a baggy. Another unique way to make the base to brew alkaline vegetable combination is a mushroom or celery broth. You would simply add mushroom or celery to broth. Tomatoes are in fact a high antioxidant however, if added in broth it changes the color. Or can be ate on sliced wheat bread with avocado spread and black and sesame seeds. Tomatoes have vitamins high in potassium and of course vitamin C. Which is a huge source for the heart. Eating plenty of tomatoes daily with a dash of apple cider vinegar and olive oil, cayenne pepper and cucumbers, you'll have a sweet and spicy delight sandwich spread.

Avocados are highly known to include a strong element of antioxidants and healthy vitamins. Again, depending on your taste buds, depending on what you can buy, and what you are going to experiment with, and I say this because my body started to experience withdrawal from processed meat food. Living independence from processed genetically modified food and meat isn't an easy adjustment food gratification. It wasn't easy to readapt my taste buds to plant- based. So, initially, I took it one meal at a time with plenty of water. Adding berries and lemon to replenish my throat, esophagus, and stomach to more alkalinity. Trying out different combinations with antioxidant fruits and adding ginger were a must. Everything needed to be highly antioxidant and organically grown.

Continue constantly eating alkaline snacks, bananas, grapes, walnuts etc. and drinking fruit in your water or an antioxidant organic drink.

Dinner I kept consistent with frying in a skillet lightly oil (avocado, almond, or olive oil) alkaline veggie cabbage, purple onions, green, yellow peppers, cauliflower brown Thai noodles or boiled rice. Light seasoning of organic garlic, sea salt, cayenne pepper, and oregano. Lightly dash soy sauce while frying for that tang on the tongue. Green onions, zucchini, cauliflower are also ways to differentiate your meal.

Friday

Friday is designed to be fun, so take advantage of this day of eating alkaline happy. In the morning have a nice, blended fruit drink. Anything of my favorite is what I typically would blend. Systemic from other times in the week, I would go back to an upscale market for ginger or turmeric shots on an empty stomach to double my intake for the body to begin with. A banana, tangerine and mango are a great combination for fiber and citrus energy. Or a ginger root organic drink.

During the day I would still have a snack of grapes, cherries, cucumber, kiwi, or seaweed. Rolling up brown rice cucumbers and seaweed is a delicious alkaline antioxidant mineral and vitamin intake. Or just a vegetable seaweed. Again, the amount depends on how big your stomach is. For instance, if you're wanting to lose weight fast naturally, I still would eat and get full of alkaline foods, and ultimately burn fat but in less quantities. The key to this is that your body is not intaking saturated fats, butter, preservatives, and meat, its only getting antioxidants, throughout the day. So that it may continue evolving into an alkaline environment, thus leaving your body with no option to find and waste the stored fat. Indeed, fitness of 30-minute cardio burns 400 an estimate of calories. Not to mention additional toning of the arms, back and legs to get a desired look would take another 15 minutes. The most important thing to remember when losing weight is the lesser your calorie intake a day the more weight you will lose. Unless you have specific genetic or injuries preventing you from adding cardio into your journey, then essentially, I for one still lost weight.

By continuing to keep my body acidic free eating no calorie alkaline antioxidants I maxed out the toxins out of my skin for s natural youthful appearance and then flushing out the visceral fat in my organs. And simply replacing my body with only alkaline antioxidants for the body to perform miraculously.

Suggestion of a blended alkaline fruit drink w/ ice for in between snack. Incorporating an organic natural grown antioxidant drink from a small business juice bar is another on the go shop stop.

I would try eating organic wheat crackers, celery sticks with almond butter as another snack. I would incorporate an almond milk drink. You'll notice shopping in the vegetable fruit organic produce section as a go to common aisle to find the most organic healthy snacks and drinks. Balance consumption of polyunsaturated and monounsaturated fats under 200 calories is well maintained in this section. Creative veggie cards in some markets are scattered around for skillet or steamed vegetable entrees.

For lunch, devour a bowl of salad with assorted greens cucumbers, onions, and mushroom maybe with a side of guacamole, avocado slices, olives and olive oil and apple cider vinegar with a side of sliced watermelon, melons, or strawberries. I continued to drink 1 to 2 bottles of lemon water moderately or pineapple juice. Organic pineapple juice is a high antioxidant that is packed with enzymes that fight inflammation and disease. Continuing to stay consistent to snacking I would eat red cherries for fun and eat walnuts on the way home. During any outdoor activities I would consume pistachios, sunflower, a few bitter apricot, or pumpkin seeds.

At dinner, organic mashed potatoes which is my favorite, green lima beans or broccoli mixed with cauliflower boiled or stemmed. Mashed potatoes are still a vegetable, no matter how many critics will say it's a starch or it contains sugar. Let me explain, you see I never could eat a raw potato yet it's a vegetable along with other vegetables that get steamed or boiled. When my jaw was fractured, mashed potatoes was my first solid source of food. I would incorporate at nights to coat my stomach. So, when I eat it after my injury it coats well with the consumption of greens. When I say greens, I mean, broccoli, Brussel sprouts, turnip, spinach, or kale. Every time, I think of mashed potatoes, I think of cauliflower. Depending on the preference of the evening I might cut up cucumber wraps it with seaweed, and avocado or sliced tomatoes with a vegan dressing. Which can be found in an upscale grocery if not, mix apple cider vinegar, avocado or olive oil, sea salt, garlic, turmeric, sesame or chia seeds and cayenne pepper) maybe tofu (recommended after 6 months of diet) to have that as a salad wrap if not in a bowl. Mushrooms is used to make plant-based meat patties. Veggie burgers grounded from mushrooms taste good with breadcrumbs, oats, green peppers, and purple onions. These are just suggestions to add to the creativity of keeping consistency of eliminating the growth of processed man-made genetically modified food from the brain to all remains in the body. Depending on what country you live in, if surrounded by bad food, traveling is the hardest part of staying consistent due to the availability of keeping perishable items with you cool. I can remember riding with my son's grandma observing her eating from a bag she had brought of different fresh fruit that required me to peel while she drove. It was such an inconvenience. By the time we got to our destination, I concluded to glance on places that serve alkaline drinks, organic alkaline fruit meals or vegetable smoothies. Whether it was an almond milk, Chai Tea almond latte or orange pineapple ginger probiotic drink, I began to consume several drinks a day on the go versus steaming a veggie & bean bowl on the go. Continuing to inhibit my body acidic free, no meat, no preservatives, no artificial flavored or high fructose endeavors from disrupting my detox.

Saturday

Take time to enjoy a fresh cup of cut lemon or lemon juice with organic ginger root pure honey in green tea. I would have a cereal of organic almond milk, wheat oats with blue or blackberries and honey sometimes shortly after drinking tea. Since, Saturday mostly is a day off, I spend this day catching up on rest, meditation and stretching. Introducing yoga is another great stress and tension relieving activity to continue the reformation to a new daily detox lifestyle. This builds your confidence and level of consciousness in the process of eliminating past unhealthy man-made eating and reflect on what you now know what to feed your body. Come to think of it, it's no wonder man made medication is needed to treat the body from man-made food.

If you're the kind of person that wants more tone to your body, like your arm's, inner thigh and back, naturally this is what you will drastically see change in shape eating this way. And of course, the prodigy of a 30-minute aerobic exercise speeds up the detox of toxins, manmade illness, and harmful unhealthy cells out the body through perspiration and shrinking the skin. Perspiration of the skin is how the body excretes out toxins besides the digestive system. Aerobic exercise can also be done riding a bike, elliptical, or if you are up to it jogging for up to an hour to reach maximum results. It's important to exercise all your limbs at once, if possible. This is what route I took to shed off the fat from underneath my skin, chin, back and inside my organs. Naturally tightening of the skin. Personally, I enjoy the exfoliation of dead cells, viruses, and toxins from my skin, it's how I maximize a natural glow and firmness. Perspiring toxin out the skin, is like a reptile that sheds old skin for fresh new skin, but only the new skin with an alkaline toxin free glow that keeps your skin ageless and internally processing of healthy oxidation in the body. Seeing the difference from eating alkaline food with cardio in between, versus eating meat working out on some protein shake convinced me I was achieving a difference. It was the youthful and younger deception of my age and skin. Don't get me wrong, compliments give us a way of meaningful self-confidence, however, the truth was visible. Seeing results licenses our perception of whether you are doing something right or wrong. Even when I see those who drink protein shakes, they look fabulous however, you can still see the difference.

Sunday

Starting the Sunday morning with a soothe blend of almond milk drink warmed or cooled. Add turmeric season, and green tea if you want to be creative. Now I unfortunately, have nothing against cow milk, again I seen better results from drinking almond or silk milk. Plus, in my case, I suffer from gastrointestinal problems, so if I were to drink cow milk it would ultimately obstruct detox of toxin out of my gut with more animal toxin. Cow milk may contain toxins or residue from contamination of whatever the cow met. Drinking almond milk or soy plant-based milk typically coats your stomach lining with rich Vitamin E, which is a very important antioxidant. Vitamin E supports the immune system by helping to protect cells from free damaging radicals. Contrary to cow milk which is notably naturally better for baby cows in my opinion. Since cows are animal drinking their milk is not a significant antioxidant in my opinion. Same goes for eggs, they are still in evolution of animal. Liquifying my stomach with almond vitamins, essentially antioxidant gently to absorb into my bloodstream reduces my chances of developing heart disease, high blood pressure and even cancer. Even if you were to have a warm almond milk cereal instead, if it is organic wheat oat ingredients with no artificial flavoring or high fructose syrup, then you're as good as green. Reason I say this, is because not all cereal is organic even when the name or caption of the branded ad composes you otherwise. You must read the ingredients on the back or side of the label where it describes the ingredients. The ingredients need to be all organic antioxidants, vitamin percentage 0% saturated fats, no artificial flavor, and ingredients and finally non-genetically modified. Trust me the organic supply is in abundance; it's just been overlooked.

Today, sorting out reinvention and combining different vegetables for alternate meals throughout the week can be tedious. Trying different salads with the adding of different seeds even if you try brown noodles stick to organic wheat non-GMO. Grow stronger to the potency of fresh organic alkalinity food and non-preservatives. Shortly after having a blended delighted breakfast of either a smoothie or avocado with cucumbers and strawberries. Since it's Sunday, I would begin brewing or planning to prepare red potatoes with either cabbage or broccoli with chickpeas in broth. Add 3 spoonful of apple cider vinegar with a sprinkle of garlic powder, lemon pepper and sodium less soy sauce. Trust me this eliminates high sodium and still giving it that bang flavor. Most of the time I would even boil brown rice in vegetable broth with a little bit of lemon juice for flavor. I prefer brown rice because it has not been bleached of its nutrients unlike white rice. Nothing wrong with white rice if it is organic. However, depending on the nature of disease, rice can make you constipated, so I stuck with brown rice. Heavy non-alkaline antioxidant season spices and ingredients are linked to cause digestive problems because it contains artificial sweeteners, GMO ingredients or unhealthy spicy spices that lead to irritable bowel syndrome. So, it's necessary to keep a maximum intake of organic alkaline spices and avoid unnatural additives and over seasoning. Basically, adopt from non-fixated inorganic ingredients to antioxidant seasoning. I would use cayenne pepper for mucous clearing, garlic and a little of sea salt helps combat sickness. Parsley flakes which help to reduce bloating and high blood pressure while supporting bone growth for a complete chef physique. Oregano season is an antibacterial fighting agent as well. Oregano is an excellent antioxidant that fights infections, loaded with iron, vitamin K, manganese, vitamin E, calcium, and fiber agent. Finally, spend the rest of the day eating your favorite salads with olives or olive oil with a splash of apple cider vinegar, or organic flavor made ready with maybe steamed or boiled seafood or tofu. Seafood is packed with omega-3 fatty acids, containing vitamins A and B, to include high in protein, less in cholesterol and calories. I left out buying a salad dressing because when I looked at the ingredients on the shelf, I realized the contents were not organic and even contained fructose syrup. Many salad dressings on the shelf contain unnatural flavor, cholesterol, and saturated fats. I would prefer the vegan dressing in the produce section if not I would make it myself. Ingredients; Apple cider vinegar, olive oil, parsley, oregano, ginger, and sometimes turmeric. Remember to refrain from bacon and chunks of meat in the salad as well, because once ingested it becomes acidic, thus resorting back to eating meat. You must think of the entire digestion of nothing but alkaline antioxidant properties. In my case, I had a benign tumor in my throat to worry about and the symptoms of Graves' Disease that could reoccur and possibly make me sick. I know many still cannot help themselves when making salad, they need meat in it. Which is understandably, a given old trickery tradition for persuading people to eat more vegetables. Again, that was the old method that I couldn't go back to. After so long of eating alkaline foods, I may only go as far as eating my salad with tofu, shrimp, or steamed/baked salmon. In the beginning, I didn't eat seafood or tofu. Moving forward, I continued eating assorted similar bowls of alkaline meals between those spikes of boredom of eating the same regimen until, I came across a different mixture. Familiarly, I fixated a mix bowl of peas, beans, quinoa, mushrooms, purple onions, and cucumber. Five years into an alkaline miracle diet, do I now twice monthly add boiled or steamed shrimp or tofu depending on how hungry I am. I concluded as to why creative meals for vegetarians are becoming increasingly popular, because when you eat a bowl of assorted antioxidant alkaline foods it gives your body a rejuvenated adjustment to even your cytoplasm, membranes, and healthy cells. However, eating the same thing sends you into a bourgeois valley. During the midst of the day, for up to an hour, experiment meditation and yoga stretching to prep for next weeks' continued transition, so you can become christened to eating alkaline foods on a regular basis. In conclusion, integrating meditation alienated distraction from modern hypocrisy and confusion to focusing on continuing down the path to an alkaline lifestyle.

THE ADJUSTMENT

Healthy foods that are naturally cut from the earth, for millions of years, traditionally were used for health, stability, and wellness for many tribes and ancestry. Indeed, during those times life expectancy did not consist of technology, processed and unhealthy fried foods. Judging from pictures of the past, there was no sign of malnutrition. Even during times of slavery, food was prepared from naturally organic grown fruits and vegetables brewed in large soups to feed a large family. Don't get me wrong, I know times have changed and the time it takes to prep and cook just doesn't fit in the normal day for some reason. Unless there's a significant other or help in the home. Cooking ware like crockpots, air fryer or large brew pots, alleviate the time it takes to make natural organic food now. For instance, it can be set on low for hours, cutting down the cooking time of being in the kitchen. Sitting the beans in water overnight into a crockpot. Traditionally, there was always a pot boiling with nutrients of vegetables was practiced traditionally throughout different parts of the world. It's an unfortunate mass struggle avoiding processed foods that has unwittily contributed to obesity or disease. The demand for longer work hours and traffic intensified fast food, quick and unhealthy meals. Yet, this is what eating unhealthy and acidic foods are in abundance of, toxins. Unless, you find an organic to-go-salad or stemmed veggie café, avoid interaction in fast food, unless it has a side of item of greens, beans, rice, salad w/no meat, mashed potatoes, or steamed veggies over rice. Ensuring the body is depleted of saturated fat and processed meat, I had to prepare my beans, potatoes, and greens overnight in a crockpot to take something with me. I wouldn't recommend cooking organic food with a microwave unless its' being reheated or it's in a steam bag. Microwaves utilize radiation to recook food, with, it would defeat the purpose of maximum results of an alkaline environment. However, microwaves are still efficiently ok to warm up prepared alkaline vegetables. If it's not over warmed. The air fryer is good for mostly all veggies except for greens. Steamed or grilled veggies light seasoning of alkaline spices with a bowl of quinoa rice, or brown wheat Thai noodles is an excellent favorite low-calorie meal to try. The noodles can be drained and topped with veggies, seasoning and soy sauce. When it's time to eat, lightly cover in a container for ultimate moisture.

For many years, the power of alkaline antioxidant food has been inevitably contained and found in organic fruits, vegetables, spices, and a high intake of water. The antioxidants that are found in certain fruits and vegetables aid to restore cellular oxidation in the bodies defense matrix. Oxidation that occurs in the cellular podium, toxins from eating meat processed, unnatural flavored, excess sugar, dead viruses, and bacteria are detoxed from the pores of the skin leaving a firm residue of a purified glowing skin.

Alkaline antioxidants attacked my issues with my autoimmune disease, my benign tumor in my throat, minimized symptoms of my acute colds, suppressed inflammation, dead bacteria, dead viruses, balancing of my vaginal secretion, preventing gastro issues and enlightened my skin. Even my anxiety and depression relapse plateaued. Over time, I experienced less and less symptoms. A rule of thumb that stuck in my head is that I didn't have to worry about no pharmaceutical substances labeled caution. Or there maybe side effects. I could overdose myself with an abundance of a natural alkalinity to enhance my immunity. Unlike meat and processed food, vegetables, and fruit, unless it appears to be molded or stale, only contains power the organs necessitate for existence.

Without alkalinity overwhelming my body permanently, I would be taking more pills for every symptom, which was harmful to my digestive system. Certain organs could shut down unconsciously as a side effect is what I feared the most taking prescription medication. But if I had to, I would essentially be mixing manmade substance with natural healthy organisms in an alkaline environment. Now don't get me wrong as I age other problems can occur, especially in my digestive system. On the bright side I can continue, drinking green tea with mint, ginger, apple cider vinegar and lemon bundled to work as a cellular antioxidant booster, working to expunge wastes out of my digestive tract and organs with no cautionary intake or label. I integrated detox as an all-day ritual. Originating on an empty stomach as the first and main hydrating intake of the day along with water. When I was experiencing constipation from taking medications before, my gastrointestinal issues expelled waste in specs and left me feeling bloated or as if I still had to go again. Now my stool, because I needed to observe with leaves my body, a natural mold of waste and healthy color, without a huge foul smell. There are different colors of our stool that tells us if there is something wrong as well. I can affirm this is not a flush that will have you back and forth to the bathroom. I mainly use number two every morning when I wake up. So, when I run, I feel less bloat. This diet isn't the same as taking a multi-vitamin a day either. However, it wouldn't hurt. Essentially, because this is allowing everything consumed to be an antioxidant or nutrient. That's what makes this diet so miraculous, it does wonders for the immune system. Even the consumption of sea moss is widely known to aid in the digestion to detox the mucus membranes from cancerous buildup. Incorporating sea moss into this lifestyle on a clock work basis is also highly recommended.

Next to consuming sea moss, is seaweed. I can literally precede large consumptions of seaweed throughout the day. Repeating high levels of vitamins with excessive skillet mushrooms and potatoes and tomatoes wrapped in the flavored seaweed. Mushrooms ultimately help prevent heart disease and is high in vitamin B which help prevent infections and helps restore cellular health. Potatoes are also full of antioxidants and they function as a fiber which is important for weight loss. When my jaw was broken, sipping on whipped mashed potatoes was a healthy source to maintain weight. It's safe to say scientifically there are significant natural organic extractions grown from the earth that deliver impeccable amounts of antioxidants for an alkaline immunity to occur. Bettering my chances of decreasing the abnormal growth inside my body. Ultimately, getting in the best shape of my life.

Pulling through

I designed a meal plan to aid in pulling through the balance with any schedule to include work schedules because of the stress of living on the move with multiple incomes. You must become your own personal coach, because mentally it is a challenge to consciously tell yourself to continue eating alkaline antioxidants. On some days when I am more tired than usual, I must coach myself, to channel out relinquished thoughts of breaking the lifestyle configuration of an alkaline diet. Let's face it life is already confusing enough, even during times of a pandemic was their conflicting confusion. Even then did I consistently consume high amounts of alkaline antioxidant vegetables, and fruit meals. When I found the available time to go to the gym to access equipment to tone my body, although was limited from a pandemic or interrupted with post injury aches, financial anxiety barriers parenting obstacles, I still had to pull through. So, I had to shuffle around times or locations to get the cardio and tone I desired. For instance, at my son's practice, if I had little time to go to a gym, I would find a walking trail safe spot to get my 30 min cardio. I had to extend my limitations. I wasn't aiming for body building if you will. However, I kept telling myself, "not give up, my organs need to receive as much oxidation as possible". Cardio is one of the best activities for the heart, lungs, and circulation in the body. Essentially, because it creates a fast perspiration of unwanted foreign damaging cells out the pores in ready for digestion. Living to see the best results of a detox alkaline diet, no matter where I was or what obstacles I had, commitment was key to detoxing for a miracle immunity to help my body fight.

In short, the most difficult obstacle of this journey is incorporating cardio. Majority of people in need of losing fat from internal organs that have health barriers will find it hard to tackle. Generally, a non-excessive workout is not as stealthy for a lot of us who have leg and back problems. If you have bad knees, back or the inability to run and jump, then a mere harmless bike or elliptical is an alternative for cardio. With this diet going to the gym to simply tone the muscle and skin by riding a bike or elliptical is still increasing the work of the heart rate to speed up the intake of oxygen in the blood to begin the perspiration inside and out the skin. So, you see the skin and the digestive system is the two ways the body exhales unwanted cells.

Since I suffered from a broken jaw, put on a liquid diet, a benign tumor diagnosis, and Graves' disease, these became a barrier for resorting back. In person, and without a filter anyone would wonder what I was consuming on a regular because of my appearance. Staying committed is the only way I saw a permanent change. Looking in the mirror to remind myself to be thankful for becoming aware of alkaline antioxidants.

There is a big difference in people who consume meat and people who consume vegetables in the way they appear. Meat engrosses longer time to digest versus vegetables and fruit for one. Secondly, truthfully speaking facts, fruit and vegetables are perishable and rich in vitamins containing infinite enzymes to revive the body's immunity. Pushing antioxidants, vitamins, and minerals directly into the bloodstream, keeping the organs functioning better with less infarct. One day you look at yourself in the mirror and notice that your slowly and steady looking less like a tired cannibal. Even I had to come to the reality that I didn't like the way I appeared, face was sagging, arms were flappy, stomach was jelly. When clearly, my immune system was desperate for restoration and rich oxidation to clear up bad radicals that were destroying my skin, body, and energy.

Some may ask is eating this way declaring to never eat meat again. It's simply saying you will have the naturalist, organic flux of toxins restored with rich antioxidants for combating disease in a disease-free combination of foods instead of spending thousands in cosmetic surgery or prescription management. Eating this way changed my whole concept when I now go grocery shopping. It's like I trace the same path directly to the same produce section as my first stop, circulating around to be creative with anything else healthy. Churning out buying cheap unhealthy food to mask budget hunger when I'm out driving. Today, there is a catalog for plant-based meals and the very best ones are in upscale grocery stores. Many have alkaline combinations in the freezer; however, it must be microwaved. I began incorporating these meals randomly after 6 months of detoxing. Some of those meals contain corn or carrots. There is absolutely nothing healthy about corn or carrots. Corn sticks to the intestinal wall. It's because they have an outer shell that contains cellulose. Enzymes are not strong to break that down. Carrots are acidic and eating too many a day lets' say over 10 carrots a day, can cause carotenemia. In this alkaline miracle diet journey, I did not include any frozen vegetables to achieve maximum filtering of antioxidants in the body either. Instead, I would buy them fresh from the produce section. After, 10 years of this consistent lifestyle my body would reject anything manmade, animal meat or inorganic. I can only imagine I would either experience nausea and vomiting or diarrhea. My tumor has not grown, my Graves' disease and symptoms are suppressed, and my overall digestive system is routinely exiting out any weakened cell growth on a natural duration. Again, some illnesses are beyond control, however, intervention is the first step to take to therapize the body.

Focusing on the positive, I became more conscience of my calorie intake. Ensuring that I was not losing too much weight I would keep watch of my weight loss as well. I continued to weigh myself and conduct a body mass index test every week. To ensure my body mass was in healthy normal range practicing self-care. As it's now a decade later, scheduled for a routine check-up after my 2012 diagnosis of a benign tumor, all my blood work came back in healthy normal range. Which is a miracle when your doctor tells you that you have a benign tumor that can become malignant, and that you have Graves' diseases and hyperthyroidism, and you will need to be on a pill for the rest of your life to now I have normal healthy function? Naturally, I also had to cut out high calories of say like a veggie burger. Veggie burgers have 200 to 300 calories and unsaturated. Yet still, I would eat that with some veggies. Unquestionably with no soda, diet soda, caffeine, pink lemonade anything with high fructose, acid, or inorganic flavors. A lot of store-bought soup in cans contain high fructose corn syrup, pork, or meat and bio engineered organisms. If you look at the back label on the nutrition label, you will see how inorganic it is. There has been a series of newly made plant- based soup no animal meat in it. Only plant-based meat. It's now wonder grocery items are being remarketed to indicate no GMO on the front or back label. The causes of GMO preservatives are causing health issues are becoming widely identified. Essentially, genetically modified organisms are grown in a lab to mimic what we should eat, without it being preserved healthy or with alkaline antioxidants from organic richness. There is even a movie documentary about GMO. Exposing the shade of the companies responsible for selling GMO. Dr. Sebi was right, to minimize my fight against life's unexpectant illness, I had to take out everything that could harm my immune system and restore it with only the best quality of alkaline antioxidant foods.

Initiating an internal armory if you will. An easier way of coping with the physiology of my body instead of not knowing what the physician is talking about. I became the asset instead of a liability. Creating a barrier full of antioxidants. Considering many of the medication that help fight inflammation, bacteria, and viruses, think of it this way, if there was a cysts' growing on your liver, what foods would you need to eat all day?

"You're taking on a challenge to better yourself"

 It takes a person to be dedicated to their body's immunity and ability to live as long as possible to continue this lifestyle. Instead of you the motto you only live once when really you must eat for your organs to live. After all we are living amongst mother nature. There are many diseases out there are life threatening, the Ebola virus for one. And even in that outbreak reportedly some people actual survived the Ebola virus. It was said that the medical staff that survived the autonomous of the Ebola virus continuously fought with hydration while sweating out the virus. In an alkaline environment, no disease can exist, however, it could simply depend on how aggressive your system is. Yet, still eating an alkaline antioxidant diet is the only research that had a major effect throughout my body. In which, anyone would seek after if they're experiencing a life-threatening issue. The only way to protect your internal environment is eating everything that will increase the body's natural defense.

Important to remember: Results may vary; however, you can expect to lose up to 6-10 pounds your first week with this meal guide. The cells in our body are designed to use stored fat for energy, especially in hard areas due to inactivity and lack of exercise. Remember the body burns up to 45 calories at rest, when fasting. Leaving cardio responsible for tightening the skin and speed up the body's natural immunity response to filter out toxins.

It just takes an overall personal desire to keep in constant progression...

GROCERY LIST

As your walking through the produce in a nice produce section here is an inventory list of alkaline antioxidant foods: Vegetables are fresh for as good as a week and a half once you bring it home. After cutting them anything unused should be sealed in separate container or zip lock to maintain freshness. Budget no more than 75 to a hundred for the week. My budget a week estimated about fifty to 100 dollars. I would spend a quarter more on occasional vegetarian outings on the weekend, if not at home.

Purified Water or boiled water in a Tea Kettle

Almond, Coconut, or Silk milk

Organic Orange juice, organic pineapple juice, organic cranberry juice, organic kiwi juice, organic

Grapefruit juice, and organic prune juice

Organic Green Tea leaves or Bags

Olive, Almond, Avocado, or Coconut oil

Tomato, Mushroom, Potatoes or mini potatoes, peas,

Organic Broth or Vegetable Broth

Organic Honey

Lemons

Apple cider vinegar

Mint leaf vegetable

Ginger vegetable

Broccoli, Cauliflower

Tomatoes

Cucumber

Zucchini

Kale

Collard Greens, Turnip Greens and Spinach

Purple or Regular Cabbage

Lettuce

Purple, white, or yellow onions depends on your choice

Sweet potatoes

Olives in jar

Red and Green Grapes

Melons and Watermelons

Bananas

Pomegranates

Pineapples

Kiwi

Apple / Green Apples / Organic Apple Sauce

Rice or Brown Rice and Quinoa

Seaweed or Sea Moss

Asparagus

String, Green beans

Bean sprouts

Green Lima beans, Black beans, White beans, Kidney beans, Navy beans

Blackeye peas

Chickpeas

Vegan Seasoning for dressing for salad (Garlic, cayenne pepper, lemon pepper, oregano, parsley flakes, sea salt, turmeric, ginger)

Organic Wheat Multi-Grain Crackers

Organic Wheat Oatmeal

Red, Black Cherries, Blue Berries, and Strawberries

Almonds, Walnuts

Pumpkin Seeds and Sunflower seeds

Seeded crackers

Quinoa

Black Seeds

Porcini mushrooms, Baby Bella, or White mushrooms

Turmeric Root & spice seasoning

Turmeric shot or Ginger Shot supplement

Tofu

Extended Alkaline Inventory

Fruits: Green/ Red Apples, apple cider, avocados, bananas, berries, melon, fruits, dates, grapes, grapefruit, lemons, limes, mangos, nectarines, oranges, papayas, peaches, pears, pineapple, pomegranates, melons, tangerines, coconut, watermelon, kiwi, and blackberries.

Vegetables: Artichokes, asparagus, brussels sprout, lima beans, string beans, beets, broccoli, cauliflower, cabbage, celery, cauliflower, cucumber, eggplant, garlic, kale, lettuce, porcini mushrooms, okra, onions, parsley, cilantro, peas, organic peppers, potatoes, pumpkin, radish, romaine lettuce, spinach, squash, sweet potatoes, turnips, zucchini, olives, tomatoes turmeric root, ginger, and sweet potatoes.

WEEK OF MODERATION

<u>**Here's a breakdown of how I tailored alkaline eating from the beginning of day to the end of the week.**</u>

<u>**Sunday**</u>

<u>Morning</u>
4am-8am 2 to 3 large cups of Green tea w/Ginger, Lemon, Apple cider vinegar & Organic honey eating later maybe a banana/sliced green or red apples/ berries wheat bread with flax seeds smeared avocado or a hot organic oat cereal with blueberries/bananas. Slither the rest with two tall glasses of organic juice ensuring cut with alkaline fruit in it or blended.

<u>Mid-Lunch Break</u>
9am-12:00pm Drink tomato soup in a cup or brew tomato soup in a bowl, added zucchini mushroom and cayenne pepper rice sometimes with cut organic fruit in a water or organic pineapple as main fruit drink/ w wheat seed crackers on the side.

<u>Post Lunch Break</u>
1pm-3pm Organic fruit in water for drink with a mushroom or potato soup, nuts and dried fruit snacks or a tofu sandwich with spinach tomato and purple onion or maybe an avocado inside.

<u>Dinner</u>
4pm-6pm Two-glasses of almond milk with sliced strawberries and blueberries to coat the stomach lining, skillet cabbage, zucchini, onion, green pepper, or spinach with a side of organic beans of choice. Or boil potatoes, Brussel sprouts spinach and onions/green & jalapeño peppers with quinoa or wheat rice.

<u>Bedtime</u>

7pm-9pm Coconut, Almond or silk milk to wake up with a fresh face and digestion, if still hungry snack on cracker.

<u>Monday</u>

<u>Morning</u>

4am-8am Have at least two blended Strawberry Banana kiwi with either milk or ice. Make it thick for a fuller filling. Wheat bread avocado, tomato, cucumber with black sesame seeds (packed with B vitamin, minerals & antioxidants) stacked like a BLT (bacon, lettuce, tomato) sandwich but the complete healthier opposite.

<u>Mid-Lunch Break</u>

9am-12:00pm Organic apples, strawberry blueberry made from home or organic blended smoothie from an upscale store. Baked organic wheat bread roll with flax seeds or sesame seeds from a fresh bakery. Wheat rice/organic beans or mashed potatoes with no gravy with asparagus or broccoli or grab a quick to go bowl of some cooked greens with beans.

These suggestions are scattered to be creative

<u>Post lunch break</u>

1pm-3pm Sliced fruit in water for drink. Organic perishable smoothie drink maybe with probiotic ingredients low calorie (under 150). Broccoli or potato soup w/ a fresh wheat bread roll. Snack or fruit of choice sliced, in a bowl or blended (Bananas, kiwi, strawberries, melons, oranges, grapes add ice or almond milk.)

<u>Dinner</u>

4pm-6pm 1 or 2 waters with sliced fruit. Skillet vegetables w/tofu or potato soup and salad sliced cucumbers, tomatoes, vegan egg, tofu with salad.

<u>Bedtime</u>

7pm-9pm 1 glass of purified aloe cucumber water, almond or silk milk, seaweed, sliced orange, or broccoli salad with dates.

Tuesday

<u>Morning</u>

4am-8am Green Tea w/ ginger, lemon, apple cider vinegar, and organic honey. Or one or two glasses of organic orange juice mixed with pineapple, turmeric season and cayenne pepper take in a to go mug. Include a banana with strawberries or a plum, with sliced peaches (not in syrup) and walnuts.

<u>Mid-Lunch Break</u>

9am-12pm Salad wrap no meat or vegetable sushi roll add seaweed and soy sauce. water bottle or a tofu sandwich with tomatoes, lettuce, or spinach.

<u>Post Lunch Break</u>

1pm-3pm Bean soup with maybe cucumbers add diced tomatoes combine spinach, celery and mushroom, broccoli, or cucumber salad. Seaweed and rice with soy sauce.

<u>Dinner</u>

4pm-6pm 1 to 2 alkaline fruit drinks with the inside of an aloe plant, boiled or steamed baby potatoes and grilled asparagus seasoning with oregano and garlic, lima beans, and rice with cut tomatoes w/ a side of a tasty organic fresh wheat bread with black sesame seeds.

<u>Bedtime</u>

7pm-9pm milk or small smoothie or oatmeal with fruit

Wednesday

<u>Morning</u>

4am-8am Antioxidant fruit in water cranberry/strawberry/kiwi or smoothie with a fresh wheat non-GMO bagel.

<u>Mid-Lunch Break</u>

9am-12pm one water bottle vegetable wrap cabbage/ avocado, cut mushrooms maybe with or without cauliflower or personal favorite bowl of those steamed vegetables.

<u>Post Lunch Break</u>

1pm-3pm Almonds or Cashews & pomegranates, berries, and grapes w/ fruit drink. Include a side of organic wheat or seeded crackers. Snack on seaweed

<u>Dinner</u>

4pm-6pm One or two tomato or broccoli with cauliflower blended drinks or roasted sweet potatoes skilled or boiled maybe a broth with kidney beans vegetable and mushroom green onions to drink after.

<u>Bedtime</u>

7pm-9pm Sliced cucumbers and wheat crackers or baked wheat bread roll with antioxidant seeds (Chia, Flax, or Quinoa Seeds). Snack on seaweed.

<u>Thursday</u>

<u>Morning</u>

4am-8am One-two glasses of milk with almonds bananas/ cashews or walnuts on the side or blend all together. Add a side of Dates as well.

<u>Mid-Lunchbreak</u>

9am-12pm Tomato and cut potatoes in a broth soup with maybe Brussels or Bean sprouts/ add peas in soup crackers on side, alkaline fruit in water with a side of wheat brown or white rice w/tofu. Seaweed on the side.

<u>Post Lunch Break</u>

1pm-3pm 1 Green/Red Apples almonds cut & water bottle or 2 alkaline mixed in water fruit drink with a snack of tofu sandwich or sesame sushi vegetable rolled with seaweed cucumber and avocado and cauliflower

<u>Dinner</u>

4pm-6pm Bowl of herbed brown with quinoa rice and black or favorite beans onions and steamed or skillet broccoli sautéed mushrooms, asparagus with a water with cut lemon & cucumbers.

<u>Bedtime</u>

7pm-9pm 1 or 2 cups of Silk or Almond milk. Cucumber and tomato sandwich with antioxidant season and vegan plant-based mayonnaise.

<u>Friday</u>

<u>Morning</u>

4am-8am Green hot tea lemon, ginger, apple cider vinegar, and organic honey, almonds or blueberries in a wheat oat cereal arranged with a side organic grapefruit juice organic honey fruits w/ green apple & kiwi blended smoothie or separated by preference.

<u>Mid-Lunchbreak</u>

9am-12pm two glass of waters with an alkaline fruit salad, or a cucumber or broccoli salad made w/ organic ingredients mixed avocado or olive oil and sprinkle apple cider vinegar on top with alkaline seasoning and herbs. Wheat or seeded crackers

<u>Post Lunch Break</u>

1pm-3pm Smoothie organic alkaline drink with a tofu or skillet mushroom, onions, green peppers vegetarian sandwich with seeds and nuts as snack. Kale green apple smoothie from home or store bought, alkaline drinks, Ginger, pomegranate, or aloe.

<u>Dinner</u>

4pm-6pm Sweet potatoes baked or steamed, diced pineapples, blackeye peas or black, kidney beans, spinach, and cauliflower skilled or steamed with sliced tomatoes organic wheat noodles and olives mix steamed or skilled.

<u>Bedtime</u>

7pm-9pm Almond, silk, coconut milk bananas/grapes or melons cut to perfection.

<u>Saturday</u>

<u>Morning</u>

4am-8am Green tea antioxidant mix. Or two waters a bowl of cucumbers with tomatoes add onions, apple cider vinegar olives, walnuts and black seeds and a teaspoon of oil (avocado, coconut, olive).

<u>Mid-lunchbreak</u>

9am-12pm Alkaline sliced fruit (melons, kiwi, strawberry etc.) in one or two waters and maybe made from home a spinach, kale, ginger blended smoothie with pineapples. A cucumber or broccoli salad or side of grapes/ cut kiwi organic wheat bread or seeded crackers.

<u>Post Lunch Break</u>

1pm-3pm 2 to 3 Aloe in water drinks or Chlorophyll algae drinks and organic honey on top of a side of sweet potatoes and pineapples with maybe broccoli or cauliflower.

<u>Dinner</u>

4pm-6pm Green tea detox mix with steamed red or regular potatoes, broccoli & olives bean broth garlic lime tofu and wheat Thai noodles.

<u>Bedtime</u>

7pm-9pm Alkaline smoothie or green tea w/ginger add organic honey or warm almond milk with green tea bag with organic honey and a dash of turmeric seasoning.

Compendium

Depending on personal preference of alkaline foods, this is just to grocery guide you on the journey of how I got started. Combining these into a skillet with healthy monounsaturated and polyunsaturated fat oil with fresh alkaline veggies. A side of boiled quinoa rice and beans became my ultimate way of keeping a healthy solid fiber base in my system during downtime. Along with healthy sliced bananas or avocados early in the morning/afternoon. My favorite luncheon, organic broth with a dash of apple cider vinegar, lemon to simmer up mushrooms together with a dash of alkaline seeds and antioxidant spices to sip on as well. I would add celery, bean sprouts, spinach or even tofu to my broth sometimes depending on my appetite. Broth to me would deliver a warm citrus therapeutic waterfall to my stomach, lessening up acid and comforting my esophagus and stomach muscle. Making me feel less hunger and fortified. Every salad with no meat. I would either buy from an organic restaurant, merchant, or purchase from produce or just whip it up at home. Ensure that you are exceedingly conscious of the calorie intake, I cannot stress that enough. Keeping it under 800 is burning lots of stored saturated fat.

One of the most misconception of weight loss is eating several meals to speed up metabolism. Which is Ludacris! Only a young soul with topflight could manage to tackle that many calories a day and still burn them. I highly recommended getting creative with combining alkaline vegetables to endure pursuit of no calorie meals, so there is none to less fat weight gain from saturated fat. No matter what alkaline food you boil, steam or skillet together decide to eat and differentiate daily, alternate it to ensure it has high amounts of antioxidant, and that it fills up your tummy quantumly. Leaving out the excess sauces and dressing like heavy season all or marinated sauces. Prepare alkaline as close to organic as possible with alkaline seasoning without man-made sauces. Even our ancestors sought out fresh foods daily and brought it back to the home. In those days' there was no such thing as a refrigerator.

Conclusion

Although individual results may vary, this 7day week moderation guide is composed of all alkaline antioxidant fruit, vegetable, and herb seasonings meals. Minus alcohol, coffee, and anything else that is unspecified as organic nonacidic in this lifestyle journey. For a decade now, I eat these foods on a consistent basis as meals. After my test results came back normal, I felt a huge relief that my circulatory system was normal. Depending on your specific preference of an alkaline fruit and vegetable, I found it easy to stay consistent by using this guide for creativity. I would also incorporate fasting during the day to reduce inflammation in the body and ultimately support weight loss. Which is vowed to support healthy function of the organs.

To say the least, it is worth more than spending a certain number of hours working out or even procuring extra health care costs for prescription management. But if you can devote yourself to a higher level of commitment, this weight loss antioxidant undraped guide to alkalinity as your body's revived chemistry is only helping your organs.

In addition, focus with meditation, by way of inserting stretching and a calmness routine for stress and mind therapy. This is a great way to cope with a healthy lifestyle change, by blocking the bad thoughts of temptation in resorting back to eating GMO unhealthy disease-causing habits. Meditation also abbreviated as a rhythm to find the energy to include cardio routine schedule, strengthening to increase the speed of weight loss in my organs.

In short, today, plant-based eating has become a very popular healthy attraction. In the past, times I was on the go, I could barely locate on the go alkaline specific foods organically prepared. It was mainly a small restaurant or family restaurant would I find fresh cooked vegetables. I would order their sides of vegetables and sometimes I would get a platter of vegetables cooked very well. When, I didn't have time to do the cooking, and the dishes, parenting, or work obligations if you can relate, buying a meal made this fresh granted me more time to relax and restore. In the late evenings, if I desired a snack it would mainly be almond milk in warm oats and with alkaline fruit. The biggest barrier I had to face was finding the time to go to the gym as I mentioned before. Especially, when

I began witnessing my weight shift slimmer significantly and not sickly. I didn't see excess f
pockets. I grew more anticipated to get 30 minutes of cardio. In the meantime, try to keep stead
of what not to consume and remember to look at the ingredients, calorie intake, sugar, etc., on th
back of anything you buy to understand where the path will take you. As the journey to detox th
mind, body and organs converts to an alkaline antioxidant lifestyle, the organs begin to perspir
naturally out toxins, bath thoughts, bad bacteria, and growth. Eating to live, thus, in the end i
what keeps the body and mind in constant quest to strengthening and fighting off disease. Caus
let's face it, our mind and health, is our sanity.